IN THE MIDST OF BI-POLAR DISORDER

YOU'LL FIND A PRAISE

Ronda Brooks Wilson
and Paul Wilson

authorHOUSE

AuthorHouse™
1663 Liberty Drive
Bloomington, IN 47403
www.authorhouse.com
Phone: 833-262-8899

Published by AuthorHouse 12/03/2021

ISBN: 978-1-6655-4542-6 (sc)
ISBN: 978-1-6655-4541-9 (e)

CONTENTS

Chapter 1   Stress Struggle and Pain.. 1

Chapter 2   What's done in Dark Comes 2 The Light................. 9

Chapter 3   Breaking Past The Pain...................................... 19

Chapter 4   Coming from Darkness to Light 29

Chapter 5   Help is Just A Call Away 39

Chapter 6   A Blessing in Disguise 53

Chapter 7   The Call is Greater then the Crisis 63

Chapter 8   Love Lifted Me.. 71

Chapter 9   Say It to See It.. 79

Chapter 10 God Did It.. 87

Dear reader, when you read this book I want you to understand how important it is to speak the word of God and believe what it says and to stand on the word and what God says in spite of the situation. Not thinking about what it seems like or looks like just trusting God and demonstrating that trust by what you do, and doing what's pleasing to God in spite of what it looks like or feels like. Then you will be operating in Psalms 34 saying I will bless the Lord at all times.

CHAPTER 1
Stress Struggle and Pain

This book is a story of stress struggle and strain a depression that everyone thought would remain but God came in as a strong wind blows erased all the madness and turn the darkness to gladness and gave me a chance again I'm not going to say first second or third chance because he is a god that gives many chances. As I can remember back to age 10. I was about 140 lbs in about 4 feet 11 inches medium build I could easily pass for 14 or 15. I was mature for my age and I thought I knew it all I didn't know why I was never satisfied only when things went my way I was a 6 grader and I was very very angry mean and upset the majority of the time I gave the teachers a hard time and I always was doing something whether it was fighting arguing or acting out, I was very outspoken by the time I was 11 years old still dealing with issues very confused I thought I already had the answers to life and looking for love in all the wrong places. I did have a few friends coming up as a adolescent there names was lisa and Valerie but as we got older we grew apart but i can remember my first church encounter with Mrs Hinton she stayed on Michigan Ave it was a apartment complex all the children would play together even her children they had curfews but she was the only one. I new that talked about church and knowing God one Sunday she took me to church I was around 11 years old. I can remember her saying baby get to no Jesus your going to need him. We all do. I didn't no then but I found out later I thank God for her anyway eventually I begin to like a young man that was the age of 17 We snuck around for about 6 months my mother and my grandmother did not know eventually I ended up pregnant, by the time was twelve years old I had to go to a hospital in Detroit because the pregnancy was in my tubes all I can remember is being put to sleep and the next day it was over not realizing years later I will always wonder about the child I never had, still having mood swings not understanding what I was going through what was going on with me. I eventually continue to stay with the young man but we begin to have arguments and disagreements by the time I was fourteen years I had abortion I had been assaulted I was mentally and physically abused but the frustration didn't stop there the wounds healed on the outside and left cuts on the inside the young man that I was dealing with he knew that whenever we got into a disagreement he would hit me so the wounds would. Not appear but he was hitting me in my body area not in my face and at that time I thought I was in love and I didn't want to get anybody in trouble. So I kept it to myself eventually as I got older I outgrew him and we went our own separate way. I can remember the last incident we had I was around 17 I was at my friends home with her mom and brother visiting now years later her brother became my sons dad. Anyway at that time I was visiting my friend. And my boy friend at that time was around 23 years old we were slowly separating he knocked on the door of my friend home. I answered that door my friend said wait her name was Martha. That man pulled me outside and begin to beat me so bad i thought I would die. But her mom came downstairs with a gun outside and said let her go. He saw the gun and ran I ended up with a broke nose. And jaw and 2 black eyes. I truly believes Mrs. Viola save me god really used her to bless me after that night me and the young man never spoke again a year later I started dating my friends brother but I still carried baggage along with me I was still hurt upset and angry and didn't know what was going on it was like I was five or six people at different times I was dealing with so many different personalities I was like a walking time bomb by the time I was 18 years old I was off and running my grandmother raised me my mother and father was always in and out of jail well prison my grandmother did her best gave us a lot of mother wit and knowledge. she also provided for us we had everything. We needed at least we thought so. She always told us the mother wit quotes you know those sayings like the grass is greener on the other side don't cry over spilled milk closed mouths don't get fed don't throw rocks when you live in a glass house yourself. I had other siblings a younger sister she was about 14 years old we called her niecy, and a younger brother named montez. He was around 16 I was the oldest my grandmother was paralyzed on one side of her body but she did her best to raise us her and our grandfather 6 months into being 18 years old I thought I was grown I thought I could go and do what I wanted I started hanging out and going to different places and parties a friend I grew up with he was a young man about 20 years old another time I considered a childhood friend similar to like having a close brother i was at a party one night and he was trying to get a ride home I felt it was harmless because he was a childhood friend, we all grew up together right before I dropped him off I can remember getting halfway to the destination to a street called Snow Road I never forget that road, I was told to pull over at gunpoint and to get in the back seat it had to be close to midnight I was raped. At gun point inside of my car after he was done I told him I wanted to get in the front seat to get my clothes I got out of the car first and he proceeded to get out of the car after me but when he stepped out I was already in the front seat and looking in the rearview mirror I drove off with his clothes and his gun in the car and left him outside the car. I went to my fiance job at the time and from there I went to the police station and the hospital, after a series of tests were performed I was back at home again lying on my stomach for 3 to 6 weeks so now I had more baggage to deal with as I said before the wounds healed on the outside but there were cuts on the inside and it didn't stop there a year later I had my first son by my boyfriend at the time that child's name was Jimmy he was named after his dad. he was the first grandchild so the grandparents which was my mom and grandmother had him the majority of the time so that left me a lot of free time to get into the fast life yes I did graduate from Ypsilanti High School in 1985 and I also graduated from Washtenaw Community College in 1989 as a computer operator I didn't have family members to help me pay for things such as tuition books Transportation you know how some young people they have parents to buy their cars pay their tuition even get their rent paid off so I did not have that, so I decided to work a part-time job through a temporary service and make some extra money on the side, one thing that always stayed the same was the stress the struggle and strain I always had emotional mood swings sometimes I was happy sad angry and mad never stable never knew how I would react I was always a roller coaster up and down so here I am in 1986 with a son and being the first grandson I was always able to drop him off at my grandmother's house the majority of the time he stayed with my grandmother. I always would leave in the morning for work for 8 a.m. to 4 p.m. I would get off work and sit with my son till about 7 p.m. then I was off and running I decided to sell drugs I really thought I knew what I was doing I made a lot of money at least it was to me at the time it was about $1,500 a week and I was able to pay my rent pay my grandma's rent and send my mother some money because she stayed in Ohio My grandmother raised my brother and my sister and me we loved our mother but she had a life she wanted to live and it didn't always include us all the time, we had a choice to go visit her wherever she stayed but we choose to stay with our grandmother we had a solid foundation didn't like being uprooted living here and living there we were not babies anymore we were young adults from my experience when parents miss out on children's childhood whether it may be abandonment or if they got sent to prison when the parents come back around it's like they're trying to play catch-up or makeup for what they miss. Once that time is gone you cannot go back and get it you are an adult and the parents still trying to deal with you like your. a child it's not their fault it's just that they get stuck in the time of where they left the child at. I was making money I kind of new drugs because I grew up around them marijuana selling drinking and smoking don't get me wrong we were well taken care of as far as clothes food and shelter we had everything we need when you look from the outside but internally I was suffering and I am sure my siblings were to especially on. the inside from frustration confusion anger and questions that I wanted answered like why were our parents in and out of prison why couldn't they get it together little did I know that it was a cycle that had to be broken but I found that out later. so now I am beyond 20 years old driving in my nice car I bought from hustling drugs going to clubs with gold rings on my fingers and gold necklaces around my neck and at this time I had a pager on my side because this was in the 80s, I did have a phone in the car which was very popular at that time handheld phones we're not quite being used, here it is my son going on 2 years old not knowing what is around the corner now I'm old enough to go in and out of clubs because I was past 21. and I joined a motorcycle club called the

CHAPTER 2

What's done in Dark Comes 2 The Light

B oogie down don't get me wrong it was like a family we looked out for each other we had each other's back somewhat more than your own natural family I also had a few friends in motorcycle club her name was dean a close friend of mine she had a beautiful loving family one time we went to visit her mom. I call her Mrs. Pearlie. l never meet anyone that treat you like family and never new you. her mom was amazing treated me like her own it was a blessing. I guess it was true they say southern people treat you like family and I got to experience it personally so here it is 1990-1991 I also had a close friend of mine we always would go out together his name was Bob he had a good heart he was a sharp dresser we work together at the convalescent home in the kitchen we were more like siblings or close friends we never was intimate together we were more like buddy buddy we both hung out for years but as time went on we grew apart because he had his own life and then with me having children I had mine as time went on we separated and went our own ways, but we stayed in touch now my son is going on 5 years old I was getting money doing what I thought was having fun, but I would soon see the results of my choices that I had made it was early spring 1991 around 80° nice outside I was going to make a drug transaction it had to be after 4 p.m. because at this time in my life I just felt like I needed more money and I was not satisfied I guess you could say I was greedy one thing about money it can't buy you happiness and it can't buy your healing my mother always told me the hustling game is quick money quick time and quick death. I met this man in the parking lot I was introduced to him by a former customer This Woman's name I will call her Ms. C. little did I know she caught a case and use me as a get-out-of-jail-free ticket this lady was like a friend of the family I would give her money to pay for her bills help buy her food and her groceries she was the last person I thought would use me to get out of jail, one time she introduced me to this man whom she claimed was her cousin I would meet up with him three to four times a week he would spend two or three hundred dollars every time sometimes he would trade cases of liquor usually she would go with me when I did a transaction since she said he was her relative we would go together but the officer need me to do the transaction alone this particular time without her. I called her to ride with me but she said she couldn't go I went on my own we met up at a store down on Packard Street down to Ann Arbor I gave him what he requested and I pulled off within 5 minutes I was pulled over they ask me to step out the car. At the time a family member was there name mr T. my grandma nephew was there the officer ask me to step out the car i was told I was under arrest, I can always remember my grandmother told me not to go make transactions she didn't feel right about it but I went anyway they took me to jail and come to find out the close friend Ms C was in my transcripts she used me to get out of jail ticket because she had a case a street name for that would be called a snitch thank God it was my first offense in the judge gave me a delayed sentence the judge made me drop a urine a I tested positive for marijuana and they sent me to a clear house treatment program the same officer that got mrs c to snitch for him was harassing me to do the same. I was confused I could not understand how can a police officer try to use you to do these things I didn't understand something like this could happen in the police system and still be legal thank God for the treatment program I was sent there and 1991 it was here I was diagnosed with a bipolar disorder a chemical imbalance which requires medication daily to live a balanced life without the medication you would be unstable have constant mood swings have manic highs and lows of depression I began to tell the clear House Representatives about the continuous harassments I was getting from the officers so I was put on lithium and prozac which I had to take three times a day since I was a property of the Clear House they were not able to harass me anymore, even though I was under a doctor's care and on medication I continue to drink I was a Wine Drinker I liked the Taste after 5 months passed I didn't go back to Selling drugs because I was on medication and under doctor care I didn't go back at that time but you have to understand that a dealer is as bad as a user the user is addicted to drugs a dealer is addicted to making the money from the drugs. That was a blessing considering I was facing 2 to 10 years 8 months pass and I got my sentence they gave me probation. Life time probation but after 5 years god delivered me off probation and within a year I was back doing the same thing again but I did it different this time I wouldl go get a lump sum of drugs and give it all out on credit and every two weeks I will go by and pick the money up from different customers. As I said before a dealer is just as bad as a drug addict is a dealer is addicted to making the money the drug user is addicted to the drugs I was under a doctor's care and I was also off of probation things got to be a little difficult for me, I managed to juggle my medication and drink on the weekends and go out. now I was beginning to understand why all of these situation occurred in my life it was not my fault. I had been battling with the condition for years but it didn't get diagnosed until 1991 confused but still drinking going out partying and doing what I wanted, yes I would go by and see my son sit with him make sure his needs were met and leave money when I had to then I was off and running after 7 p.m. knowing that my pill bottle said no drinking no alcohol because the medication was not to be taken with alcohol I was in denial about the disability and the condition I was diagnosed with some days I was happy sad confused upset quick temper. I had some days when I spent too much money made bad choices I was out of control I found out this is called the manic stage then I had days when I wanted to just give up with suicide thoughts little did I know what was around the corner I will get up at 11 a.m. and check up on my grandmother because now I did not have a job I was diagnosed with a disability with a steady income I had income and I was still on the drug scene making money I had a few Associates one of my closest friends her name was Pat my fiance's cousin and I also had Yvette which is his cousin also and I'm not going to leave out my uncle his name was Corky he passed away, we would all get together and play cards drink and listen to music now when we had the card games Yvette would contact our forth player Doug we were all like family. sometime we played at Yvette's house or sometimes at Pat's house .we would have a good time but Pat was my running buddy. We talked about everything we drank we hang out and laugh sometimes we just got together and just a rode all day laughing and talking but I always knew on the weekend we would meet up at either Pat or Yvette's house and this was also a way I made a few dollars on the weekend, but I was still on medication and I was drinking and as they say what you think is hid in the dark eventually will come to the light. Here I am 26 years old but I was having the time of my life still not taking this condition seriously I ended up pregnant with my second child here It is 1992 all the while drinking became occasional and taking medication was adjusted to a mild antidepressant my son was born May 12th his name was James thank God I wasn't drinking and I was token off antidepressants before he was born I thought with two kids their father and I will be together now, he had two sons you know the fairytale dream and our relationship will get better which we did get better for about a year after our son James turned 2 years old and Madness started again me and their father had trust issues so much had taken place in my relationship with drinking drugs and sexual relationships with other individuals that we didn't trust each other me being still on medication didn't help because when I did drink on the weekend I became very paranoid by the end of 1993 our relationship had ended we still remain friends I was dealing with the bipolar disorder and also he wasn't trying to be responsible father right now you know how it is when you feel as though you have time and you want to hang out we both had some growing to do by the time James had gotten to be three and Jimmy was nine, me and there father separated went our separate ways he still would visit the children every now and then our oldest son Jimmy mostly stayed with my grandmother I think from everything I was going through and not taking the depression seriously it was kind of like a pressure cooker I had so many things cooking in my mind and in my thoughts that it overwhelmed me, and I ended up cutting my wrist and they put me in a Saint Joseph Mental Facility 4 to 8 weeks and the sad thing about it I had to leave both my children in the care of their grandmother all the while I was detain for 8 weeks having different mood swings very emotional because now they were trying to stabilize me on medication and it was like I was on a Merry-Go-Round and I need to get off but I didn't know how the cuts on the outside of my wrist healed, but I still carried the scars on the inside that never healed it was just more baggage added to what I already was carrying around with me when I was released after eight weeks I tried to drown out my pain by drinking and going back to the motorcycle club again my drinking and going out had got better because I had to take a look at my children and start being more responsible so instead of staying in town whenever the motorcycle club went out of town on the weekends I will go with them I would leave my children with their great-grandmother she always knew that when I got back in town me and the kids father would end up having disagreements so I started going out to cabarets I also was a regular motorcycle Club member so whenever they went out of town I went, but it was mostly on the weekends because I did have a part-time job through a temporary service in 1994 I met a man whose name was Paul but before I met him I almost got married to a truck driver named James thank God I didn't God intervene in that situation see I found out people that deal with bipolar disorder have highs and lows and ups and downs and sometime you just up and do things without thinking spending money making bad choices display out of control Behavior so you have to be careful. I thank God that year I didn't get married and the man that I met was a Christian in church and I was considered a bad girl off-limits I was not in church I like to go out I like to drink and I like to party I was pretty nice looking on a scale of 1 to 10 I think I probably would have been about 7 or eight. I love to wear low-cut skirts every weekend paul would get out of church and come looking for me at his cousin's house, we will be there partying and playing cards and just enjoying ourselves it was the weekend so he will come with the intention in mind I'm trying to invite us out to church, but I had other intentions sometimes I would there until 1 or 2 a.m. my children will be with their grandmother, at this time my mom was in prison she had been off and on back and forth to prison all my life I was told she'll be coming home soon, one night while walking home late at night I just stayed through the pathway across from his cousin's house he wanted to make sure I was safe he had good intentions he wanted me to get home safe but I had other plans because I had said previously I was a bad girl one particular night after we met it was around July 28th 1994,yes I did have a vehicle but I played like it would not start, so as usual he walked me home and one thing led to another, and we ended up going out as far as the church goes after a few months he relapse into bad ways which is called backsliding which means he was in church at one point but he went back out into the world, I was sad for a minute but what happened after dating him had to be a setup from God as I said before I was not a church person he was we begin to go out August of 1994 after his birthday I still continue to go out on the weekends mostly to visit his cousins I was on medication prescribed by the doctor but I hid it very well as the old saying what you do in the night will come to the light, still taking medication drinking maybe on the weekend not everyday I didn't realize that what I was doing was causing Paul to want to drink and do things also eventually after dating Paul for a year he began to use drugs and our mother was released from prison at the end of 1995 she lived with my grandmother in the same apartment complex that I lived in so with me drinking and having access to drugs everyone expected me to give them drugs including my mom, I began to leave the drugs alone because our mom was home and she was using my fiance was using but, I was not on the street selling drugs but I became the one that would give it to my fiance so he had access to it drugs all the time I began to drink more and still take the antidepressants I would go to work at 5 p.m. and go to yvette house at 8 p.m. and stay till around 2 in the morning and as I said before my kids will be with their grandmother at this time, my fiance was on drugs my mom was up and down the street on drugs after being released within a year so here we are going into 1996 the early part of it. The New Year had already came in everyone was excited after February because it was income tax time people have money to spend I found out I was pregnant with my daughter. Her father name her Jessica. Finally a girl I told myself she will be my last child. My mom was excited because she was a girl since I already had two sons my doctor practically took me off the antidepressant I stop drinking after the third month begin to take care of myself and eat right and get the proper rest but in the seventh month I had high blood pressure from my last two pregnancies with my too son I was always diagnosed with toxemia its a condition in pregnancy also known as preeclampsia characterized by hypertension a sharp rise in blood pressure leakage a large amounts of protein into the urine and a swelling of the hands and feet and face by the 7 and a half month I went in for a checkup and her heart was not beating the doctors rush me upstairs to the emergency room because they could not find a heartbeat .as I look back it is very sad how the enemy is able to manipulate our minds in order to prevent us from focusing on what's important as I was getting prepared to lay on the ultrasound table the first thing that crossed my mind was to call my number Bookie and to see. If I can get my numbers in before 7:15 and then to contact her dad second I notified him and told him I was at the U of M Hospital and they were about to take me in for a C-section because they couldn't find a heartbeat this was at 6:30 p.m. Jessica was born at 9 p.m. that night they removed her from my abdomen but she was not breathing they ended up hitting her on her bottom two or three times and she began to breathe her heart rate was beating again she was born October 28th

1996 Jessica AnnMarie my moms middle name but she was diagnosed with fibular hemimelia fibular hemimelia is the shortening up a fibula at Birth for the complete lack of therefor Jessica had a 3-inch difference in her leg one leg was three inches shorter than the other and the doctors could not treat it at that time until she got past three years old but she was a miracle baby because she came into the world and she wasn't even breathing and didn't have a heart rate after our daughter was born my mom's drug usage got worse she was drinking more and doing more drugs her plan was she wanted to take Jessica back to Ohio but her and Jessica's Father Paul had many disagreements he was not going to allow it. I had told my mom no its to soon but her dad standing 6 feet 3 inches went to my mom and said no my daughter cant go and that was it .his drug usage slowed down after Jessica was born he got himself a job because he had more responsibility especially with his other two children that he had in another

CHAPTER 3
Breaking Past The Pain

Relationship my mom became very violent not to us but to others on the street she was very militant rambo-style she would wear a long black trench coat and she would carry a machete strapped to her leg she was diagnosed with schizophrenia and looking at her you couldn't tell she was diagnosed with a mental condition she was about 5 foot 9 inches and weighed about 150 lbs, she would put you in the frame of mind to Pam Grier, when she drank she was very Bodacious and out-of-control I can remember in 1997 watching her walk down 1st Ave and pour gasoline all over her body and light herself up with a match while I stood about ten feet away from her I ran up and put the fire out and she was admitted into a mental hospital after being treated for 5 months she was back to drinking and doing drugs again, same program once more you couldn't tell her anything late 1997 and the middle of August I can remember taking off of work and going to the doctor with my mother Dr Brooks he told her that she has six months to live she was diagnosed with cirrhosis of the liver which comes from drinking and the doctor told her that she replied if I'm going out I'm going with a bang I couldn't believe what she said she didn't even consider her own children or her life I had no words to describe how I felt all the way driving back home that day not understanding how she didn't care about her life or leaving us. I didn't know whether I was angry hurt sad it was so many emotions I didn't understand after that she went back to doing what she always did drink and smoke as I said earlier our mother was not a sloppy Drinker when she drank you cannot tell she didn't slur her words she did not fall over she would get upset when she ran out of drinks, to look at her you couldn't even tell she had a drink when ever she did take one. I had a part-time job so I will leave in the morning at 9 a.m. on my way to work I will leave my kids with my grandmother everyone else is in school except Jessica she was about one years old at the time I will get off work at 3 p.m. get home by 4 p.m. her father would have her he will go to my grandmother's house and pick her up this is around June 1997 it was warm outside 70 or 80° everyone was enjoying themselves until 8 p.m. or 9 p.m. especially since school was out that I was able to go out more because the kids didn't have to go to school in the morning so I can go to work and didn't have to wake them up I was able to leave them with Paul after 12 noon he would take the kids down to my Grandma we stay in the same apartment complex 5 minutes walking distance summertime me more freedom didn't have to get the kids I did my visiting in the projects at my friend Yvette house was where everybody enjoying themselves and probably listen to music play cards my oldest son Jimmy enjoyed it because he was able to come with me she even had children his age when the weekend was over I have regular doctors appointments every two weeks at CMH mental health for regular check-ups for medications to make sure I was taking the medicine they made it where I had to get blood drawn so they can monitor the medication level I was not a smoker so I didn't have to worry about them finding traces of drugs in my blood and the wine was out in 24 hours so why not drink with cheap wine Wild Irish Rose Mad Dog 20-20 Boone's Farm basically I can get a fifth of that bottle for $5 I like to drink for the taste I would get a little paranoid but that wouldn't stop me because it was the weekend I was off work it was my way of relaxing and enjoying I thought only God knew what was lurking around the corner the following year here we are coming into 1998 as they always say new year new beginning 10 months later no one could have prepared me for what I was going to experience next I was still on medication but I was taking it properly had the time I was taking Prozac because I had been on a number of different medication since 1991 such as lithium Wellbutrin Cogentin Etc but at this time it was just Prozac I'm hid it pretty well from individuals I didn't want anyone to know I was taking medication here we are going into my 1998 at this time my brother in and out of jail he made some bad choices but my mom was not much help in the area some things she encouraged but that is another story after me I was still trying to find myself now having

3 kids including my daughter everyone still drinking going out on the weekend I was still leaving my kids with my grandmother my oldest son Jimmy was 12 years old my middle son was six and my daughter was 3 years old stayed with my grandmother a lot during this time but Jessica and James was with me and Paul until I got off work through a temporary service and my shift was 7 a.m. to 3 p.m. Monday through Friday on the weekend I still went out and visit my so-called friends also decided to make a little extra money on the weekend since everybody was always looking for drugs we played cards on Friday and Saturday and I will go over to a friend of mine's house and we did what we had to do on the weekend it was our way of relaxing and make my extra money on Monday came we went back to our old same program going to work getting the kids out to school taking care of things to the week I'm looking forward to the weekend me I was still in denial still hiding medication drinking alcohol on medication my mom was staying with my grandmother so that did not make things better my mom had started doing more drugs she visited her friends and Associates when she did them during the day she will come back home at 8 p.m. to my grandmother's house and we could tell by her behavior that she was under some type of drug influence she was frustrated and angry when she didn't have money for drinking and drugs and she would threaten our grandmother most of the time I ignored her unless she seemed like she was out of control as if she was going to raise her hand. every morning my mom had a routine she would get up every morning at 9 a.m. fully dressed sit at my grandmother's kitchen table and and wait for the liquor store to open at 9 a.m. her favorite drink was Colt 45 and a half pint of Smirnoff what she had to have at least three times a day to her it was like breakfast lunch and dinner don't get me wrong our mom was a functional addict she would take a bath and wash up cook dinner she still function daily I can remember particular month around early May 1998 my mom was trying to buy some drugs on the street and she got into it with a young man she was

known in the community for taking people's money and pulling guns the man went to make a sale to her at 7 p.m. she hit him and there he hit her back her intentions was to Rob him she came home and we see she had got into a disagreement and talked about what she was going to do to the young man we took her to the doctor because her jaw had a lump in it from her struggling with this young man that would not go down so we took her to Beyers Hospital and upon examining her they found out she was a diabetic and had to be put on insulin which is good for diabetes but. the bad thing was she was a heavy drinker when she was released from the hospital she was upset but we did find out that she was a diabetic if that incident hadn't occurred with her and the young man we would not have known about her condition so basically I can say that because we found that out we did get some extra time to spend with her because she slowed down that drinking but the drugs got worse and even though the situation took place what the enemy meant for bad God has turned it around and use it for good. God was working through the young man and brought our mother more time to spend with us because after we found out she was dealing with diabetes and she began taking insulin the drinking kind of slowed down it went from three times a day to maybe one or two times a day we would ask her not to drink and not to do drugs because when a person is dealing with diabetes when you drink the alcohol and it gets broke down in your system it will rise your sugar levels really high which is also dangerous for a diabetic but that didn't stop her at all she still continue to drink regardless of her condition me I still worked took care of my kids while continuing to go out on the weekend even though I wanted her to take care of herself I still had to take care of myself I had three kids I had to provide for I will still take an antidepressant mild antidepressant Wellbutrin Prozac but I was still in denial about my health and my condition this was a daily routine for me that went on for months now we're coming up on the month of September and which my mother and my sister both have birthdays my mother never really asked for much on her birthday she always wanted to cook lasagna and garlic bread that was her favorite for everybody to come by and eat I find it when you have a parent or parents out of the home due to incarceration or whatever the issue Maybe there will always be issues concerning the child and the parent you will find that the parent will always be trying to make up for what they miss and the child will always deal with abandonment issues I think because our mom miss so much of our childhood she always thought she can go back and get it but once it's gone it's gone at times she would get upset at our grandmother because our grandmother had a lot of memories with us and she didn't because she was always incarcerated this also became an issue because they would have disagreements she felt as if our grandmother was taking us away from her and it wasn't that it was just that we were all grown up now we were now adults and she wanted us to depend on her but we had our own lies and we had to depend on ourselves and what we were able to do not at this time my brother was incarcerated and my sister was trying to move on with her life my younger sister Denee she is very sensitive we call her Niecy she was very smart & a computer wiz she always had her child hood friends they were always there for each other Carmen Miko Shanova as she got older then came Denecia Tameka. Sharonda Monique and her friend from work Megan they always had each other back as for me. I was the oldest my focus was family & keeping things together and being the oldest a lot of stuff fell on me. Not that I. Had to but its how we were raised especially responsibility of taking care of everyone which included my brother he was incarcerated and going back and forth to jail me and my younger sister had to keep money on his books anybody that have family members in jail they would know about that my grandmother also needed help and I also had my own family I was determined I didn't want my children to go through the things that I went through I did not know how to stop cycle but I was determined to do whatever needed to be done to help my family. They were all I had a lot of @responsibilities fail on me which caused me to try to handle more things then I should half mentally I was not able to but I thought I could it got very difficult thank God Paul was in my life now after my mom's birthday everybody was still a little frustrated because our brother was not there he was incarcerated in spite of the situation we were determined to keep the family together as time passed we came into the months of November this was the month of giving thanks and Christmas is right around the corner my mom still did her same routine of getting up every morning around 9 a.m. getting her alcohol set up for that day her favorite drink again was Colt 45 and a half pint of Smirnoff but this particular morning November 15th 1998 our mom was not feeling well she was a little worried about my brother because the next day November 16th he was supposed to be sentenced to 15 years around 8 p.m. my mom began to complain of a headache she wasn't feeling well my grandmother called me and told me to come to see about her I arrive at my grandmother's house around 9 p.m. I stayed about two minutes away and the same apartment complex I knew my brother was being sentenced to next morning November 16th me and my younger sibling Niecy but we still had hopes that he would make it home but my mom was very frustrated that night she just kept saying over and over I don't know if I'm going to see him again I tried to comfort her and tell her mom we are going to appeal this case we all knew that they said he was facing 15 years and it was very frustrating I tried to get her to go to the hospital but she refused she took a Tylenol for pain and I sat with her until 1 a.m. she said she was going to lie down and that was a long night for me I kept in contact with my younger sister and I let her know what was going on I went home to my house and I tossed and turned and I couldn't sleep I woke up all through the night I saw any minute my grandmother will call and ask me to come take my mom to the hospital I lay awake until 4 a.m. I finally fell asleep and woke up the next morning knowing that my brother had to be sentence about 1 pm. I went down to my grandmother's house after I got my children out to school I got there about 8:30 a.m. I wanted to check on my mom whenever I went to my grandmother's house my mother was always sitting up at the kitchen table but at this time it was after 8:30 and she was not sitting there so I asked my grandmother where's my mother she replied she was asleep still in bed I proceeded to the bedroom to wake her up when I got to the room I saw her under the sheets covered up my mom was in bed and she was really cold and very stiff there was no pulse I began to say Mom I began to shake her but there was no respond I called her name but still no response I went back to the living room and told my grandmother that she's not responding my grandmother with a strange look on her face said Ronda bring me my child my grandmother didn't have a phone at that time so I pick my mom up and carried her and laid her on the couch in front of my grandmother my mom wait about 150 lb and I brought her into the living room my grandmother said she is the last of my my 10 children my grandmother had a hospital bed and she wasn't able to move without any assistance I laid her on the couch and went to the rental office next door as I was racing and running and sweating and breathing heavily somehow deep down I had already knew I told the assistant and the workers in the rental office to call 911 I then went back to my grandmother's house no one was there except me and my grandmother the kids were all in school Jessica was still at home with her dad when I got back from the Rent office I told my grandmother 911 is on the way I still begin to check for a heartbeat and a Pulse my grandmother kept yelling saying she was the last of my 10 children waiting for the ambulance I sat there but deep inside I knew she was gone she was too cold and unresponsive the paramedics came within 15 minutes but it seemed like an hour they laid her on the floor and they began to do CPR but I can hear one of them say she didn't make it at that moment I was more concerned for my grandmother because of her health condition and that was the last of her children my mother Patricia Ann Brooks the ambulance took her to the hospital I got my fiance Paul to sit with my grandmother while I went to the hospital time was passing it was soon after 10 a.m. and I knew that my brother was going to be sentenced at 1 p.m. the same day I was on my way to the hospital with my mother but I felt numb it was like I didn't have no emotions I couldn't think of what I was feeling I was moving but I couldn't feel any emotions it was almost as if it was Unreal on my way to the hospital I managed to contact my sister as we enter and told her we was at Beyers Hospital and it didn't look good my younger sister was really sensitive whenever we dealt with circumstances and situations we had to be

CHAPTER 4

Coming from Darkness to Light

Careful how we told her and I didn't want to tell her too much over the phone because I didn't want her to get so emotional that something would happen to her on the way to the hospital. as I sit there and wait for the doctors to come out and my sister to pull up the doctor came out at 11 a.m. and pronounce our mom dead as I stood there in the hospital it seemed like there was nobody else in the world but me when my younger sister came to the door I looked at her and she knew but at that time all I can think of is what am I going to tell our brother when I arrive at court at 1 p.m. he expecting to see our mother along with us so I told my sister to go sit with her grandmother and me and my husband went to Circuit Court in Ann Arbor I begin to tell my younger sister I'm going to the courthouse he is expecting someone to show up and she did not want to leave the hospital but I told her you have to go back and check on her grandmother so she sat with her me and Paul headed down the highway to I-94 Ann Arbor Circuit Court it was about a 20-minute drive when it seemed like 2 hours all type of thoughts began going through my mind what would I say to my little brother or even to the court what would happen to our brother how would he respond with the judge let me talk to him questions after questions and thoughts after thoughts heart racing and I began sweating once again can remember walking in the courtroom thinking about what I am going to say when I get in a courtroom it was bad enough that he was being sentence but how could I tell him this heart-stopping news I said Lord give me strength I opened the court doors and the courtroom was full of people I saw the judge Melinda my brother was standing next to podium with his attorney I asked attorney if I can speak with our brother I told the attorney that our mom had just passed and I wanted to address the court to let my brother no as they began to tell the judge she began to reply this is too much of coincident the young man's mother passing an hour before his sentence they acted as if I made it all up to slow down the court proceedings I asked if I could tell our brother before he was sentence they gave me a few minutes in the court and as I began to tell him about our mothers unfortunate passing he began to take his fist and hit the podium in harder and harder and harder when they told him he was sentenced to 15 to 40 years in prison he still hit the podium. So hard as if he never even heard the sentence after it was over he looked at me and said losing my mother is for Life 15 years is nothing compared to losing my mother they took him away after that we said our goodbyes held each other with tears running down our face we told each other how much we loved each other I told him we're going to appeal this case I left the courtroom my kids begin to come home around 3 p.m. so I need to get back home James is in the first grade Jimmy was in the sixth grade I had to explain to them what was going on Jessica was too young to understand that was a hard matter for me because I had much to do things had to be prepared such as funeral clothing picking out a funeral home who would attend the service my mom didn't attend the church none of us did it this time. this was a wake-up call for me my grandmother couldn't do much because she was paralyzed on the right side brother was headed for prison but they did let him see our mother before he went off to prison for hour without any family members my younger sister couldn't do much as I said she is very sensitive she was there and that was enough for me so as usual the majority of responsibility fell on me I knew I had my work cut out for me I didn't know Jesus then but I know I needed help now I began to miss doctor's appointments at CMH I began to slack off taking my medication I also had a amazing case manager whose name was c. Wilson, I did not tell them my mom had passed they had no idea what I was dealing with my grandmother didn't want anything to do with the funeral proceeding she didn't even want to attend she looked at me and began to say Ronda you're the oldest and you're going to have to take care of everything I had to set up the funeral I didn't know who to go to or where to start but I did remember getting my hair done at a place called Hallelujah and there was a pastor there named Pastor Davis I went to this pastor with tears in my eyes and asked him if he could help me with the funeral. He agreed to do the eulogy so from there me and my sister began to pick out our mom's clothing, earrings, and I was tasked with styling her hair. It took everything in me to comb her long black hair. I did her hair and I gave the funeral director her clothes for the burial service that was being prepared I really needed to talk to my therapist because I was emotionless it was like I was running on some type of energy I couldn't explain as I said it didn't even seem real I had no feelings at the time I think I was more angry then hurt I felt like our mom was selfish and wasn't thinking about us because the night before she could have gone to the doctor she could have went to the hospital but she refused it was determined that the cause of death was a diabetic coma I could just remember her words I'm not going to be here to see my son do 15 years in prison that was a really hard time for me specially dealing with depression taking medication there with my kids and little did i know four years later I will come across the same situation. after everything was over the funeral service and the families went home you are all alone what's next now you have to pick up all the pieces and go on. I was not even coming in for. blood draws my grandmother began to get concerned for me my daughter was set up to have surgery because of discrepancy in her leg that she had when she was born they were trying to set up for an operation by the time Jessica was 3 so now I had a lot of work cut out for me. Jessica is 3 years old James was 7 Jimmy was 13 years old James quiet and stay to himself and was very intelligent Jimmy was determined quick with his hands and loved his music Jessica just the regular 3 year old that laugh and giggle together with her brother .but with our mom gone you never forget its certain things that remind you of them .the food they like to eat the perfumes they used to wear how they wear their hair the conversation they used to have the kids would asked about our mom. but I had to talk to them at the same time I needed somebody to talk to me I was not responding to doctors I didn't want to talk to anybody I was going out drinking and hanging out late I was leaving my kids with their great-grandmother not realizing that she may have been going through to she was also the last of my grandmother's 10 kids. as time went on I talked to my therapist and my doctor because my behavior got worse but for the sake of my kids I open up to my counselor and confided in her I told them what I was dealing with, and that was anger frustration they began to adjust my medicine and get me back on track but I was working off and on through a temporary service I also receive disability so I didn't have to work much Now here it is going into the year of 2000 Jessica is now 4 years old James is 8 years old Jimmy is 14 years old I have been in church for a year-and-a-half my mom died November 16th 1998 on the same date our brother was sentenced to 15 years in prison within a year my stability was deteriorating I can remember it was December 5th 1999 I was invited to a church by my hairdresser her name was Minister Boone the church was called Cathedral of Deliverance The Bishop's name was Bishop Watson I had not been in church and over 20 years I was in my early thirties my grandma knew I needed help so she sent me to find Min Boone. but she told me she would know exactly what to do next. I didn't know where to look for her at it was about 3 p.m. and I decided to go on Ecorse Road to Taco Bell I enter Taco Bell in place my order it was a gas station I pull to the gas station to get some gas and there was Minister Boone coming out of the gas station with a pop in her hand it was too much of a coincidence I begin to tell her about the situation with my mom and depression and how my grandmother wanted me to locate her she invited me to her hair salon next door which I had no idea about she began to tell me about a church and the following Sunday I met her at that church I got baptized December 5th 1999 and my life was never the same again everything I thought I knew was a lie after being baptized I was filled with God's spirit and my life changed for the better I begin to read the Bible and renew my mind with the word of God my favorite scripture was Romans 12 verse 1 and 2. I beseech you therefore brethren by the mercies of god that you present your body a Living Sacrifice holy and acceptable unto God which is your reasonable service. i new my mind had to be renewed. by the word of God by exchanging your thoughts for gods and doing things the way the word of God says not the way you want to do it. because if you can change your thoughts you can change your life I began to go to church Sunday school a year later when Jessica's Father Paul Wilson started attending the church all three of my children also begin attending church I begin to enjoy the teaching and understanding things we're coming together I began to have peace and a lot of things that I used to do I didn't want to do any more the more word I received and meditated on the less I wanted to have anything to do with the things in the world my oldest son stay with my grandmother the majority of the time but he would go to Youth Development on Tuesday with the young people as the years went bye I began to deal with health issues it was around May 2001 when I got sick and went to the hospital I was told I had a brain aneurysm and at that time I suffer from severe headaches it was treated with steroids and it was corrected all the time I would be throwing up and I would have to be put in a bathroom I was in the emergency room at least twice a week but I still went to church at the end of 2001 going into 2002 my health begin to get better I knew that I wasn't drinking and going to parties anymore I made up my mind I had to loose my life for Christ for the sake of my kids and myself I always said that meaning I had to give up the world and everything pertaining to it. And receive the word of God and serve God I began to read the Bible twice a day for 30 minutes to an hour I attended Bible study children's church and church service on Sunday people would say it didn't take all of that but it did I need a new life and a new way of thinking and it had to be changed and I knew it was not going to be overnight I didn't want my children to go through the things I went through with or deal with the things I had dealt with I wanted something better for them and I know deep in my heart that Jesus was the only way to get it. I didn't know how much but I knew that if things are going to change God will be the one to do it. So it was all or nothing at. all .now this is the beginning of 2002 New Year's Jessica had already had one surgery on leg the doctor had informed me and her father that she would need three or four more surgeries by the time she was six I knew my work was cut out for me. Jimmy was a teenager I was determined he was going to make it James never really was no problem he was quiet and stay to himself my brother was still incarcerated our dad also and I knew if I was going to make it. it was going to take Jesus he was the only one that was going to do it so I began to read the word of God I began to pray and to tell the doctor that I was in church and the Bible studies in the word of God was helping me. after being in church for 3 years my medication lessen the doctor begin to take me off the medication because my mental stability was improving I was happy and making progress I even took my grandmother to church twice in a wheelchair paul was still using drugs all the while i was in church. But i prayed and he started attending a little more me and Paul got married April 10th 2000 in Lucas County I knew I couldn't live in sin and I wanted a change he was attending church on Sunday with me also. My son Jimmy got a job at Meijer and I continued to go to church take medication study the word of God because I knew the only way I'd make it would be through the word of God. As time went by I began to get a plan and work the plan. I began to look over my life and everything I had been through and also other individuals that dealt with the bi-polar disorder health condition, suicidal thoughts, losing family members and financial issues. I realized that other individuals had support teams. They had their mothers, fathers, aunt, uncle, other relatives to depend on, but all I had was my three children and Jesus. My husband had his own health issues and his mom and dad was still here, but in every situation in my life all I had was Jesus. It is true that he will never leave you and he will never forsake you. I came to realize that he was there even when I was not thinking of myself, he still loved me and kept me. Through it all I realized that it was the word of God that changed my life. I began to look up healing scriptures, **Psalms 103:5, Isaiah 53:5, Isaiah 26:3**. Whenever I got frustrated I began to meditate on the word of God because I came to realize that it was the word of God that had delivered me and set me free.

Not only that I understand if I take care of God's business he will take care of mine. I also thank God for the convalescent home ministry that was started by Evangelist Conerly and Deacon Conerly. After 2006 when the Conerly's moved on in the ministry and the Convalescent home outreach ministry was turned over to our outreach team at the Cathedral of Deliverance. Our outreach team would meet two to three times a month at the convalescent home where we would minster to the elderly. This ministry was truly a blessing to us. One thing I learned is you should always be a blessing to others because you never know who may have to look after you. When you bless and look after others you're also being a blessing unto yourself.

CHAPTER 5
Help is Just A Call Away

B ut little did I know what was around the corner 6 years later my grandmother begin to deal with a health condition she was already paralyzed on the left side but I thank God she did her part when it came to raising me and my siblings when we were children everyone told my grandmother Miss Juanita to put us up for adoption me and my siblings but our grandmother refused to divide us up we all graduated and attended College for years I always heard that we were the children that was not going to amount to anything that we will be, criminals like our parents but my grandmother believed God anyway she had a stroke February 2002 that It was very difficult we took her to the hospital me and my husband and my sister we were told after a couple of weeks there was nothing they could do me and my sister decided to take her home the hospital wanted us to put her in a nursing facility we said our grandmother took all three of us when no one else would. When no one was there for us she was and now me and sis which is what we called each other was going to be there for her. We didnt have much but we had love so we decided to take her home and we begin to take turns feeding her and care for her as usual but by March 2002 she had had another stroke she couldn't say much the nurses recommended we put her in a hospice and me and my sister was there everyday along with her friend Penny my sisters friend Penny work in the medical field so often time she would come back and forth to hospice to visit our grandmother we were told that we didn't have enough medical experience to assist her my oldest son Jimmy was really hurt because the majority of his time was spent with his great-grandmother at this time he worked at Meijer he was going on 16 years old he had just started working I did keep him informed and talk with him about his great grandmother and her situation my brother was calling and I also still had to attend church one thing I found out even though we go through life's ups and downs life doesn't stop so you still have things you have to take care of you know how they say when it rain it pours well it was pouring time I learn thru my experiences that God won't put no more on you than you can bear. God said it in his word and he cant lie. between going to church and bible study our brother and our father which was incarcerated and getting my children to school my doctors appointments begin to decline my medicine had lesson but I still had doctor's appointments to go to but I was not going I told them I would pray and communicate with God after 2 weeks worth of no-shows I spoke with the counselor and inform them that I was well and I stay in prayer a lot talking to God Thru life experience I have learned to run to the throne and not to the phone I need god to help me and strengthen me for what I was about to face around April nineth I got a call from hospice informing me and my sister to get there to the facility we made it there about 11 a.m. our grandmother couldn't speak but she could move her head yes or no we both wanted to know was there something we could do she loved to watch the movie Dirty Dancing and she like to watch the video breaking Electric Boogaloo because the young man in the video looked like our brother we put that movie on for her me and my sister said she wants to talk to our brother or hear his voice so what I did I called the prison and spoke with the counselor told them the situation and asked could he call us and gave them a date and time and we will be available it was around noon time we didn't get no response the next morning we came to hospice about 10 a.m. by lunchtime or the 10th of April our brother called I told him the situation we put the phone to our grandmothers ear she smiled he talked to her and whatever he was saying all we knew that she was smiling after he was done I spoke with him and told him we will be up to see him and how much we loved him and informed him what was going on the next morning we came up to see our grandmother me and my sister and Paul we were there maybe an hour I told her grandma you did a excellent job raising us montez will be fine we're going to do whatever we can to get him home I also told her we loved her and we knew she was tired I also reassured her that I was with God now and serving him and that he would take care of us and that she can get some rest cause we will be okay my younger sister just laid on her chest this was around the 10th of April we all left and went home and did what we normally do that night I had a dream she got on a boat like a mayflower we were on one side waving all the people that past in her family was on other side. it was like she had to make a choice what side she wanted to be on with her living family or the family that past away. she look at me my sis and brother and waved good bye said she did her part shes going with her family we were watching standing on Dryland so the next morning me and my sister had a similar dream hospice called around 10 a.m. and told us to get there as quickly as possible when we walked in we felt and knew at that moment something was wrong .we were in the room maybe an hour I we told her we love her and she closed her eyes and went to sleep and she was gone now I had to tell my children which was the most difficult thing especially to the oldest child Jimmy because he spent so much time with her so I knew we had a lot to get prepared for and this is where I was going to need God to strengthen me. The women we knew as Mrs Juanita (grandma), so loving and caring that wherever she was you had a place to lay your head. Throughout my life I have only had two young men I called God brothers which was James (Mug) and Laronce (Roast) they were like family My grandma loved mugg. laronce. came in after she passed away After my grandmother death, Mugg took a 1,000 dollar down payment to the funeral home for her services. He loved grandma and lived with her for 10 years. I knew we had a lot to prepare for because there was going to have to be another funeral but I thank God and I gave him the praise. I was in a better place now then I was then when my mother passed. I was serving God and he was my help and my strength. I belong to a church and I didn't have to search for a pastor so I thank God for that. Everything went well the funeral was set up and it all took place we buried her on her birthday April 17th 2002. After the funeral we had to start preparing to get her apartment taken care of. We had to decide what things we was going to put in storage and the things we were going to get rid of. One nothing I found out that when there's a funeral that takes place life don't stop and just keep going on. I was really concerned about my brother because he didn't get to attend any funeral services but at least with our mom he was able to come sit with her for 4 hours at the funeral home. He was in Washtenaw County when she passed this particular time when grandmother passed he was incarcerated in Jackson, Michigan. prison. Afterwards we all went out to see him to encourage him and work on getting him home right along with our father. After a week or two of getting the apartment cleaned up three months later we moved into a house. I just don't think any of us could bear to look at the apartment anymore; it was like having a new start because within a year my oldest son gave birth to my first grandchild. Her name was talayshia. My grandmother always said when one life go out another one comes in so I told my brother it's time to get back on point with the Outreach we was doing in the facility he was in because everyone needs to be saved so me and him began to work right along with my husband Paul. Several years had passed we were still serving God and praying for our brother and after much prayer our brother came up for parole but he was dealing with health issues as well. We would talk to the counselor where he was incarcerated when we were informed he was diagnosed with blood cancer. So I began to write Jennifer Granholm the governor of Michigan at that time and the Lansing parole board and within 90 days of writing these letters I received a phone call I was informed that our brother will be home within 6 months so I thank God for prayer because prayer will go where you can't go but that was just the beginning of his health problems. He was released in December 2012 one thing I found out is that man can lock up your body, but God holds the key to your spirit. When he was released he was paroled to me.

My brother had a tendency even at 42 years old he would play with his grandchildren riding up and down the street on bikes acting like a spring chicken when he was old crow we all have sibling that act as if they have no care and no worries that always has something to overcome from relationships to females to drinking you name it he was a handful and still is I got to the point that me and my little sister begin to refer to him as the brother now that he was home and parole to me he had health conditions that needed to be taken care of he did not want to listen to anyone so we got a second opinion through the U of M Hospital it turns out that he had had an enlarged spleen even though the prison that told us he had cancer but he had a form of blood cancer where his body make too many platelets we all know when you're dealing with health conditions people can do what they want to do but when you have to follow doctor's orders you need to obey. But not Our brother he always want to do things his way. he was a people pleaser he always knew everything and sometimes he even thought he knew more than God. This is when we would often run into conflict because nobody knows what God knows. in the situation and all I could do was pray one thing I found out is that the enemy will use people you love and the ones close to you in order to get to you I can remember taking him to the hospital in 2013 one day he stood on my porch and he begin to Hemorrhage from his nose ears and other parts of his body we could not do anything except for rush him to the hospital we got him to the hospital st Joseph. all we could do was pray for me and my husband he was somewhat conscious and in the room with him was me my husband and my little sister they began to do a procedure on him to see what was going on when they start the procedure he begin to have seizures back to back causing his body to twist and turn and various ways his heart stopped for 3 minutes and they called a code blue call for the doctor to come in to resuscitate him I had to step out the room and they indicated to me that the condition is serious and he had to be flown to U of M Hospital when he got to U of M he was unconscious I was the first to arrive so they called on me for decision in regards to his medical condition he was not in shape to make his own decisions since he was unconscious me and my husband and my little sister begin to pray because I've known over time that prayer will turn any situation around the doctors came in told us he had to have his spleen removed it was enlarged and that it was crushing his internal organs causing him to bleed internally I was his emergency contact so I understood that if an important decision has to be made I will be the one who would have to make it I found that it's hard to make a decision when it comes to your own life but it's even harder when it comes to making a decision for someone else's life you don't want the burden on you for a bad choice that's made and the one whom you made the choice for doesn't make it even though he was unconscious. Me and my sister made the decision to remove his spleen yes we talked it over with his two oldest daughter's but to spare his life We decided for him to have the operation and after 8 hours of surgery when he was brought to recovery the doctor informed us that he had a condition called myelofibrosis it is when the blood produces too many platelets normal platelets are range to 400,000 people with this condition are able to make up to a million platelets and when the number gets that high it can lead to heart attacks and strokes and seizures our brother had already had two strokes and 1 heart attack so we took this very seriously before being released he was on a ventilator for about a month we all got together and prayed as we always did and posted scriptures all over his room 1 scripture was Isaiah 53 verse 5 also Psalms 103 and verse 5 we began to trust and thank God in advance for his healing I found that when you're dealing with situations such as this you can't allow anyone to infiltrate your space or your thoughts because you want to keep positive atmosphere you don't need negativity you have to have faith field individuals not negative Neds and Nancy's negativity hinders the results. in this situation you can't go by what you see you have to go on who you know one thing about me and my husband when a problem arises we come together as a team we have to be in agreement in order for our prayer to work within 3 months God had delivered our brother and he was able to come home upon being discharged we had a long road to go. but we knew that God will be with us every step of the way he couldn't remember the simple things such as using ATM machine going to the store picking out items you need he couldn't even take his medication properly he didn't even really know who we were he needed someone to assist him so the family had to come together especially me since he was living with me and my children and my husband he also had chemotherapy treatment things are very difficult for him at this time because as I previously mentioned he wanted to do things the way he wanted but he couldn't he was under a doctor's care and he had a U of M case manager so he needed things done in accordance to a schedule he had to have therapy and he had to be taught how to do things all over again due to The Strokes and seizures he suffered he wanted things to happen quickly and in a hurry and in his way but this was a process God would have to get him through all we can do is pray and encourage him to trust God he is not the god of one chance or two chance he is the god of many chances he has Mercy on whoever he chooses I will just encourage our brother and tell him if God did it once he can do it again but the question is do you believe it even now he's doing much better he still has his ups and downs but I am thankful God turned his situation around and brought him out. We still communicate with the brother everyday me and my sister and keep him in our prayers and I thank God 4 text messaging because sometimes he had to be remind to take his medication and his appointments thru a text. we still refer to him as the brother All we could do was pray, I just got so much to thank God for I truly know it could have been worse or went in another direction as my husband always say it could be worse so I learned to thank God where I'm at on the way to where I'm going because in all things we are to give thanks according to 1 Thessalonians 5:18. And as time went on I learn to praise God in every situation because I know for a fact God will never leave you or forsake you. this one may go Mama may go daddy may go sisters Brothers aunts and uncles and Friends but God will still be there we always walk away from him but he is always there to accept us back with open arms as time went on I learned to pray more and talk about my problems less I learned to tell my problems about my God and not my God about my problems because he sees all and he knows all between me and dealing with my own household and being power of attorney over our brother situation me and my husband still did God's work in spite of it all we still continued Outreach Ministry two times month with the convalescent home and we would go out and pass out flyers in the community I found out that it's not just about you but it's about who you can help to when you going through you have a strong desire to show others that the same God that delivered you can deliver them to we also begin to make a prayer box at home we would put notes inside and prayer request from other individuals than me and my husband would choose a special day of the week to pray over them within a year-and-a-half God begin to answer prayers in the prayer box around 2015 the chemotherapy treatments for our brother had became less they begin to give him pills instead of the chemo my daughter was about to graduate around this time which was truly a blessing because the doctors told me. And my husband when our daughter was born in 1996 that her legs may have to be amputated and by the time she was nine years old she already had 8 surgeries and all I can say is God is good and God Did It Again the doctors told us she would not walk across the stage to receive her diploma but June 2015 our daughter graduated and jessica walked across the stage and received her own diploma on her own two legs when the doctor wanted to amputate her legs at 4 years old but we begin to pray me and my husband and said not so. we choose to believe God and I give all the glory to God because I understand doctors come practicing but God come healing I can truly say that God changed my life and my family's life also I can go on with Miracle stories of Christ and the Miracles he has performed in my life now that our daughter had graduated it was going on July 2015 she was looking for a job. God bless her in less than 60 days she wanted to take a year off and save her money and work and make a decision as far as college after the first of the year that was fine with me it was just a blessing that she graduated God did bless her with a job it was not what she wanted but she had a job sometime he don't give us what we want but he'll give us what we need I thank God for the small blessing as well as a large ones here it is going into the end of the year 2015 this is after September 2015 me and my husband have been serving God over 15 years we found out if we take care of his business he will take care of ours now that our daughter is working and our son James had a second job one thing about James he's never any problem he loves to work and stays to himself and goes to church my mama nickname him little man and the name fit he was like a little man very responsible my sister called him Manny because he was very mature for his age similar to what they would call our father his name was Joseph but they would call him grownie because he was a grown-up for his age anyway I knew my children were blessed but James he was a special assignment he just desires to work go to college and church he has always been about taking care of business we sometimes referred to him as a little big brother I thank God for setting him apart like that our mom gave him the right name Lil Man even though now he's standing 6 feet tall it fit him she said he was very responsible at a young age then we have their older brother Jimmy and music artist he is a factory worker Jimmy he is multi-tasker like I am, always busy if he wasn't selling cars he was Selling Houses but he always made sure his mom and dad had whatever they needed right along with James. Then there was my godson Jamaal him and his God brother stay busy my godson is kind of quiet and somewhat a loner and at times he would have a hot head. He was just serious and business minded and people didn't know how to take him but he always was there for his family. I also had two step children Paul and Nikyta they lived in Lansing they mostly stayed to themselves but James Jimmy Jessica and Jamaal they were always around Ypsilanti area with us and Jimmy and

Jamaal had their own homes Jessica and James were with me and their dad but, they have been talking about moving but they had to save their money, now between me and Jessica's Dad we had to Drive her back and forth to work Jessica had not gotten her license yet, so we were pretty busy between dropping her off at work and picking her up, I also had a part-time job we still did outreach work in the community twice a month and thanking God for his strength daily because if it had not been for the Lord on my side I don't know what I would have did. I would have been like a sinking ship without a sail a lost ball in high winds. Because it's God that keeps us not ourselves for me I find that I had to communicate with God daily and thanking him for the strength that he gives me each day, sometimes I begin to look at the things that I had to juggle and when I look back over my life I've always been in a multitasking situation when you're juggling two and three things at one time I guess you would say multitasking the mess or you would say M&M but one thing I know that God can take a mess and make it into a miracle there were times I had surgical situations going on my husband had health conditions he was dealing with, and also my daughter going in and out of the hospital and on top of that dealing with our brother's health condition and him being incarcerated and the majority of the time everything fell on me everyone else in our family was decease at this time so as I said before I had to continually stay in prayer, so God can strengthen me between pharmacies and doctors appointments I can remember when our brother was going through those health problems in 2013 I was writting Governor Jennifer Granholm while he was incarcerated trying to get him a medical release so he can come home but at that time our daughter was having surgery and I was just getting back on my feet from a medical procedure See in 2007 after I had second brain aneurysm. I want you to see when your trust and confidence is in jesus he will strengthen you to overcome. Any situation God healed me after about 8 months but I begin have sleeping issues not realizing it was sleep apena our younger brother had got out of jail after a few years. He brought a young lady back from California after a visit with a family member. now me and sis always called him the brother because he was always going through something and the majority of the time he thought he knew everything anyway he end up going to jail on a violation again and he left a young lady here and I'm going to call her Ray Ray she end up staying with me and the family she started going to church she got a job

CHAPTER 6
A Blessing in Disguise

Ended up going to College but in the process I had a health condition I was not aware of one night she noticed that I wasn't breathing so I end up having a sleep study I found out I was diagnosed with sleep apnea and every 30 seconds I will stop breathing the doctor set me up for a surgical procedure because they had gave me 6 months to live within 2 months this procedure was a success but I had a long road to recovery being that she ray-ray stayed in the home she helped prepare meals and made dinner for everyone for months and I say that to say this you never know who God is going to use to help you or vice versa that's why you should not look down on nobody but this young lady (Ray Ray) was truly a blessing to our family because Paul also had health issues too. I never would of known when our brother left her here in Michigan we would be a blessing to each other. And even my son Jimmy at that time he had a young lady he was dealing with I will call her Kiki her and Ray Ray became good friends and they both were such a great support team for me at this period in my life and I was support for them. Because we continued to pray and read together so you never know who God is going to use to be a blessing to you I can remember saying Lord If I Only Had another person in the family I could call to assist me, at that moment I heard in my spirit your help is just a call away from then on in I have learned to call on Jesus not just in some situations but in all things. I learned to thank God for the little trials as well as a large ones because even though things we go through it seems like we're in a dark place at times but one thing I have learned that the enemy can paint ugly picture but when you know the artist you can always change the scenery and I thank God for staying connected staying in position to hear what God have to say because it's the enemy job to bring chaos and distraction and confusion to have you so discombobulated and now you're disconnected and we all know when you're disconnected you are in shut off, so I learn Acts 17 and 28 that its in him I live and move and have my being so the safest place for me is in him. In the eye of the storm the storm can be around you, but it don't have to be in you now we're coming into the end of 2015 around November 2015 Jessica just had a birthday in October 28th me and her dad decided it's time for Jessica to start driving she needs to get her license she took the driver's test first time without studying so she didn't do well so she made up her mind that when she go back she was going to study for 30 days and that's what she did she study she went to work and me and her dad was praying we took her to the Secretary of State that morning and we let her stay there over an hour when we came back she was standing outside waving her test she had passed oh boy we thank and we praise God because that mean we can get a break she can drive and she's over 18. She already had been saving her money and her older brother got her a car me and her dad we were home free Jessica was driving and taking herself back and forth to work she begin to get more hours on her job that was a blessing for all of us, now we have come into the new year 2016 we thank God for the new year you know how everyone always saying fresh start new beginning it coming up with all these New Year resolutions I don't believe in all of this and all of that I just believe in serving God and that's what we did me and my husband we continue to keep a schedule Outreach continue to go to church. There were times we would call Outreach for everyone. To join in but sometime people work and they do other things but that don't mean you have to stop. God's work has to go on, so what am I saying they'll be time you may have to go alone and do what God put in your spirit to do you have to be obedient and do what God say do me and my husband begin to pray and we start preparing our self for the spring and summer months ask God to give us Direction on what to do we thank God Jessica was driving now because we can make more plans to do more things in the community especially in the months when school is out here it is beginning of April me and my husband had been dealing with a situation with his health, because the doctors diagnosed him with diabetes years ago but it's their diagnosed not his we just trust God believe the word speak the word confess the word that's our part I know you can remember when I spoke up earlier about M&M. Multitasking mess now here it is after May 1st, my husband had to have a surgical procedure such a coincidence when you start making plans to do something for the Lord the enemy will try to get in but you still have to have a made up mind my husband had to have a surgical procedure we were told that he had a blood infection in his body but thank God for his healing power it didn't spread to his organs it just stayed in his big toe. his toe had to be amputated my husband is a strong man he stayed in the hospital for about a week I was there by his side after being released I had to give him antibiotics for so many days and was praying all the while because I had to give it to him through a IV but like the word say I can do all things through Christ who strengthens me now my husband have made it home and it was well into the month of June, after everything was over now we were coming into our church appreciation months we began to pray and ask God for ideas and plans but little did we know what we were going to have to face within the next 60 days but God knew he knows what's around the corner when we're looking straight ahead but I thank God for being in his word. After prayer around June and July 2016 I received a phone call from the Richard Handlon Correctional Facility which is a prison in Jackson Michigan. Our dad was incarcerated in and under doctor's care but because he was dealing with a mental condition and he was not able to make proper decisions for herself when I got the call I had no idea because I hadn't heard from our father in over 7 years yes I knew he was incarcerated he went to jail in 1983 he took $12 but he end up staying in there over 30 years I manage to write him and in the early years I used to go visit him but within the past 7 years I was dealing with a number of other situation with family such as Hospital surgeries doctor's appointments and also myself having surgical procedures. So when I receive this call from his case manager this particular day it was totally unexpected the case manager begin to tell me what Our Father was dealing with that his Health was declining and he had a cancer diagnosed and kidney issues and that they needed me to become his Guardian to give them permission for surgical procedures and treatments of course I said sure I will become a guardian, after the paperwork came back I was his power of attorney I had to make decisions for him because he wasn't capable of doing it himself. I had so many things going through my head at that time because I still somewhat was dealing with my brother situation. Me and my younger sister, and she is so sensitive I didn't want to stress her out but at least he was coming home. So I began to inform the caseworker to send me the paperwork for our dad. She told me that once it was approved I will receive the letter in the mail and the sign it, and then when they received it back I would received a letter in the mail stating I was his Guardian over the past six or seven years every now and then I would write the parole board in regards for our father but no one ever told me that his health was in this bad of a condition I began to ask that case manager how come no one got in touch with me before now why was his health allowed to get to this point but I didn't get a respond within 60 days I received another call our father had been moved to a hospital in Jackson called the Duane Waters Hospital he was diagnosed with kidney condition and his colon had ruptured and he had a cancer diagnosis. He needed emergency surgery and his condition was life-threatening I began to inform my siblings my younger brother and sister because I know decisions had to be made even though I was the guardian I still want their opinion our father was sent to an outside hospital because Duane Waters cannot accommodate him because of the seriousness of his condition I can remember after becoming his Guardian all type of thoughts was going through my mind and one thing particular came that is something when you have to make a decision pertaining to your own life but it's even harder when you have to make decisions over someone else's because what if you don't make the right decision and that's all that kept going through my mind this time was crucial and I really needed to hear from God after they moved him to the outside hospital I just started praying and fasting. I think at that time I was going to church I had to have two phones I had my regular phone in my pocket but I also had another cell phone because being that I was in one place and I was a guardian and he was in another city and state before they can do anything they had to always get my permission so I had to have that phone near me so I can respond I can remember sitting in church and they called the phone doctor's told me they would have to do this procedure and it got to the point where I kept jumping up answering the phone and then I had to let our first lady know what was going on because the procedures they were doing they had to get my permission before they can accommodate him you talking about staying in prayer I had to stay in prayer 24/7 I can remember October 15th 2016 I remember them calling me saying his colon was ruptured and it needs to be repaired I gave them permission to do that procedure after talking to my siblings. From 12 noon till about 5 p.m. and he came out of that surgery okay, but then they turn around and contact me back by 6 p.m. and said they want to prep him for another surgery the following day he had to have a colostomy and with his age they didn't know how the outcome would be doctors informed me that he lost a lot of blood and he wasn't a young man he was over 70 years old so all I can do is keep the phone next to me and pray the next morning which was Monday I went to work they call me at work told me everything went well I thank God for that but he had to be in intensive care I begin to thank God in advance because they said that they didn't know how the outcome was going to be overnight and I was not in position to check on him because he still was in intensive care in the prison many of us know when you are in a particular trial the enemy will apply pressure he would tell you or try to tell you whatever he chooses to build strongholds in thought process and strongholds are wrong way of thinking but we have to be just like Jesus in Matthew 4 and 4 that enemy wants us to doubt the word of God but I have learned that when the enemy tries to bombard your thoughts according to 2nd Corinthians 10:4 and 5 you can't go by what you feel you have to speak what the word says that it is written, that man shall not live by bread alone but by every word that precedes from the mouth of God what am I saying you have to align your thoughts and your words with the word of God and what it says in every situation you have to choose to believe God regardless of what it looks like or feel like I Choose to believe God and you begin to rest in the situation and not stress and God can manifest a blessing in your life as I said it before I learned to tell my problems about my God because God already know about my problems after my father was in intensive care for 3 days it was around Thanksgiving 2016 me and my husband begin to contact the case workers because we were inquiring about his condition but what I was told was totally a surprise the voicemail was left on my recording saying that she was sorry that our father did not have any rights or any privileges and he could not have any visits and if he wanted visits he would need to write the warden himself and send the letter to Lansing my reply to her was I was his guardian and he did have rights and in the condition that he was in he was in intensive care he didn't know whether he was going to make it or not that I should have been able to come visit him but she still replied he would have to write a letter to the warden I could not believe that the prison refused to let me see our father so I did what she asked him to do because he was not in condition to do it I begin to write a letter to the warden explaining my situation that was going on and that I was his Guardian and he'd had a surgical procedure and I wanted to visit him and I was denied visitation rights and I needed to write a letter and that is what I was doing I understand that God knows our hearts and he understood that I wanted our father at home I did not get a response in regards to the Warden but I did take the Liberty to write the parole board I begin to work with a program called friends of America that helps with individuals family members that are incarcerated, the young lady who assisted me was named Mrs. Holbrook whom I'm grateful God allowed me to meet. I filed a complaint with the ACLU in regards to them not letting me visit our father and I just believe God stepped in and took over because by January 24th or 2017 I received a letter saying that Our father had a parole hearing and I knew God was working one thing I found out that God is working even when we don't understand even when we can't see it he is still working you just have to have faith and believe .when me and my sister got the letter saying our father was to have a parole hearing we hadn't seen him in over 8 years I can remember talking to his case manager in the past when I would check on him they would say that his memory was not well I had seen him in the past 8 years but my siblings my brother and sister hadn't seen him in 20 years so the day we were going up to Jackson prison and finally get to see him God had made a way out of no way. my sister was so nervous she kept asking do you think he gonna know us do you think he's going to remember us I just kept saying I believe he will. that was the longest 45-minute ride I had been in all the way there she was asking me questions I was asking her questions but I just believed that when he saw us he will recognize us in spite of what the doctors had said one thing you find out in life and in the midst of your mess god will bring a blessing out of any. Situation regardless of what the circumstances we have to find something to praise him for knowing God gets all the glory and to praise him in every situation. Even when I felt like nobody is there or care understanding that god will never leave you or forsake you. So my job is to believe and trust god will do what he says. I might not have what I want but I got what I need. And that's Jesus so I learned to thank God where I am at on the way to were I am going, because Jesus didn't give up he made a way for us to have what ever we need as long as we tap in and stay connected. And I thank him for it, now we're driving up to the prison big giant Gates all around to visit our father I had a few butterflies and I know my sister was nervous. She just kept talking asking questions I think it was just the unexpected or not knowing we did not know what to expect but we hope for the best, as we got to the counter took out a identification the guard ask for his name because he was in the hospital part it took them about 30 minutes to get his information together I don't know why maybe because he been in prison over 30 years we sat down and we waited after she took her ID they told us they will bring him out. We sat there and looked at each other me I was praying and then as I looked up 8 stairs I saw two guards pushing a blue recliner and I can see a glimpse of some gray hair and I told my sister I think that's him right there her eyes begin to open up and we got

CHAPTER 7

The Call is Greater then the Crisis

Ready to walk up the stairs as we stood at the gate after they put him in the room we can see through the glass window they checked your ID and walked us in he looked at both of us he had a gold tooth in the front of his mouth which was very surprising because it's the same gold tooth that we remember when we were children my sister started crying I kind of tensed up I didn't want her to see me cry I'm known for doing that holding my tears I can't let it out I got to talk to him I just got to ask him one question and we both walked up to him I kneel down eye level and I looked at him and I said do you know who we are it took him about 3 or 4 minutes and he said yes you're my kids and I smile I said who am I because I couldn't believe what he just said I said sis he remember us then I said that who am I while my sister was in a corner crying he said you my oldest Ronda you the baby I delivered. And then he said the strangest thing he said God is going to use you to deliver me. tears begin to roll down my face and I walked away my sister came over there and hugged him, she was just laying across his lap I said see sis he know us he didn't forget and, then he looked up at me and said did your brother make it out of prison our dad had been in prison for so long time our brother did 15 years in prison he didn't even know he made it out I said yeah Dad he made it out and you will too I kneel down and told him do you believe God is going to bring you out first he didn't have anything to say he just said I just been in here so long and then he said yes. I do. and I said that's right we on the same page God gonna bring you out of here just believe along with us they only let us visit for about 35 minutes but we was really happy to see him I really was happy for my sister I thank God he was able to recognize us especially my sister he always refer to her as Denise we call her Niecy she mostly stay to herself she had a few friends but she was that little sister that did the traveling going here and there she had a college degree but she still had that loss of that father. We both did and its many individuals going thru that now and just cause a father in the home you can still be lost in the house.

I thank god for a heavenly father amen. So I was mostly happy for her that she did get to see him I knew God was working. My younger sister on the way back she says sis what are we going to do I said God already doing it. When I got home my husband and I sat down and talked for about an hour I told him I'm going to begin clearing out the spare room I think it was about 72 hours pass. God woke me up about 2 a.m. and I told my husband our father will be home by Valentine's Day I did not know how but I knew God was going to do it, I just didn't want our father to leave or pass away in the prison system even if he came home for 2 or 3 weeks I asked the Lord to let him come home with his family so we can laugh and talk and lavish all the love he deserves on him he had over 28 great-grandkids he had not even laid eyes on and nine grandkids he hadn't even seen my son was the oldest Jimmy which was named Joseph after our dad every other day I began to clean out the spare room packing up boxes throwing stuff out I didn't know how I was going to get the bed and the items that was needed but me and my husband just made the decision that we was going to believe God so since we said we believe God we demonstrated by what we did so we begin to get Walkers and wheelchairs and clothing we had a TV room it wasn't a large space but it was big enough for our father around February 3rd 2017 it had not even been 10 days since the visit the social worker contact me and said they awarded our father his parole and he will be able to come home to my address or I can wait 2 to 4 months so they can get him in a group home she gave me a option I told her I would rather for our father to come home as soon as possible and that's what he did I thank God for the extra room in the house after 72 hours someone from the parole system came to my home it was his parole agent he ask for me and gave me the date he said your father will be home on Valentine's Day and that was confirmation that God did what he said he would the parole agent also informed me that our father only had 4 months to live which was a surprise to me but I just thank God he was coming home, now here it is February the 5th

everybody is getting prepared setting up the house, calling for doctors getting everything in place it was just a miracle we can't believe it after 33 years our father was coming home and that was only the beginning, of the next 3 months what we were going to experience I can remember that day Valentine's Day morning about 6 a.m. me and my husband and my younger brother who went down the highway on our way to Jackson to the prison took about an hour we got there like 7:30 a.m. and checked in as usual like me and my sister did but this time we wasn't coming to visit we were coming to bring him home. We informed the warden that we were there to pick up Joseph Brooks what should have been at the most an hour. It was a three hour wait at first they kept relocating him then they didn't know where he was at I had got to the point I said I don't think they even thought we was coming to get him he had been incarcerated so long, my brother stayed in the prison waiting I went out to the car because like my sister he hadn't seen our dad in 20 years. After three hours pass I begin to call the social worker and informed them that we had been on the property over four hours and we were wondering what was the going on around 10:30 we begin to see the guards roll up we pulled the car up our brother sat outside they brought him out in that same recliner that we saw him visited in. Our my father had a smile on his face that will brighten up the world it is an unforgettable smile I never forget it. me and our brother put him in the car as my husband drove down the highway yes they gave us medicine they gave us Ensure drink and they gave him a change of clothing but as he went down that Highway our dad look at us he said I would like a piece of Kentucky Fried Chicken. Now we all just laugh and gave God the glory as we drove down the highway it seemed like we got there really quick to Ypsilanti as we entered into Ypsilanti our father began to notice how things had changed the places that we stayed on Michigan Ave was no longer there. They had been built the Eastern college and as soon as he got the chicken we ordered 5 pieces of chicken as soon as he got the chicken he began to eat Non-Stop.

I believe he ate at least three pieces and 7 minutes when we got home we made it to the house we had to get the wheelchair out we had a sign up to see, It said home sweet home we put him in the chair and sat him in the living room it took us a minute to get him up the stairs but we made it, as I begin to make call to let individuals to let them no we have made it home, I just knew someone will come by it was about 1:30 p.m. I made a few phone calls again soon, very dear friends of our father's one of their names was Carissa this was a young lady that he grew up with him and every time I went to go visit him he always spoke of the Collins family which was a wonderful family in Ypsilanti Michigan that was spoke highly. Of and two particular individuals which was. Sister Carissa and her sister Delphine they also had a sister name Marie our father didn't remember much but he remember most of his childhood friends and especially the Collins family. And when ever I mention there names he would begin to talk communicate which was a blessing I was able to talk to sister Carissa because in the town that we live in she often came to visit my church home which was her father-in-law church, and she would ask about our dad they hadn't seen him in over 30 years but sis Carissa always was able to tell me childhood. Stories. About our father and that was a blessing. I knew our dad had family but I really didn't know how to get in touch with them. and I knew they were going to want to see him because it had. Been at least 25 years since they seen him and we had not been in touch with each other either. I think the last time I saw them I was about 25 years old and now here I am over 50 so what happened I had my son go to the internet to try to locate them yes I know their names first and last name so I figured everybody is on the Facebook now so my son found one of his siblings and he left a number for them to contact us I think it took about 48 hours for them to get in touch with me and when they did. I informed them that their oldest brother was home they were so happy they didn't know how to take it they didn't come over right away but they took my phone number my address and they informed me that they would be there within 24 hours in the meantime we had a lot of things we had to set in order because of our father's health condition. Thank God we was able to get the wheelchairs the bedding and undergarments that he may need but we still needed many items he had a colostomy there were bags that he needed and supplies that he needed I didn't have a whole lot of knowledge about changing the bag but thank God for Google I understood that it needed to be changed every so many hours and he also had medications he had to take we had a nurse setup but at that time she had went on vacation so for the first 7 Days me and my children and my husband had to maneuver on our own, during the course of the day here it is after 3 p.m. I knew people would stop by especially his grandchildren and great-grandchildren he had over 28 great grandchildren he never laid eyes on I was pretty busy that day as we begin to get everything set in order 5 p.m. came around and it's one thing about our father he loves chicken he began the request more chicken, then my younger sister came and she brought food also she specifically asked him what he would like at one point he started naming off all type of food hamburgers chicken fish but we had to start out slow, it was truly a blessing to see him eat we took pictures I mean he really ate that week he enjoyed himself until I had to start paying more attention because I'm sure he wasn't used to eating this way so I had to get him set up on a pattern a daily pattern a breakfast lunch and dinner it was truly a blessing and even though he was home we still have to continue our daily duties going to church, doing Outreach just doing the things that we do daily so whenever me and my husband went out to the convalescent home we attended church services we would have my younger sister or brother will come by and sit for an hour or so until we came back, We all know the situation may change but God's work still have to go on .after about a week or so his siblings got in touch with me and wanted to know could they come by our home to see their brother. I begin to tell them yes and gave them the address it seemed kind of strange but I can do all things through Christ who strengthen me. my younger sister didn't take it that well I think she was kind of nervous she didn't know what to expect but neither of us did but I know the right thing to do was to let them see their older brother .which was our father so I set up a time after church on Sunday for them to stop by and see him he had already had his own area and room I took a few pictures I began to take pictures of everything sometime my children would get upset and I will tell them these were not just pictures these were miracles after about 30 days had passed our father had been home 30 days we had a few difficulties at first but once the nurse got set up and would come by twice a week, and we got a system set up for him with medication.

CHAPTER 8
Love Lifted Me

To be tooken and routine meals being served it all worked out. he didn't want the nurse them to give him a bath that was something I had to participate in but it was still a blessing in that, you no one thing I thank god when your stay connected. He will. Keep you 2 steps ahead. I always. Say we look straight ahead god see around the corner. Thank God that me and my husband had put a few dollars aside because of our father's supplies got low we tried to sign him up for a couple of programs one program will try to sign him up with Social Security they turned him down because he had been incarcerated for over 30 years so a lot of supplies we would normally get we had to purchase ourselves so we all had to come together even more, but we didn't mind. neither did the grandkids because this was a great miracle a lot of people have wrote Our Father off as decease but God has the last say so. now that we begin to get things situated here it is about 5 Weeks Later two big boxes came to our home they sat right on the porch they were items from the prison when my husband pulled up he began to tell us that they were some boxes on the porch, we brought them in the house and we begin to go through the boxes now that it's time to get in touch Detroit Free Press i got in touch with. Them the free press wanted to start coming by communicating taking pictures and talking to our father. As I said earlier in the book I begin to work with friends of America also there was a particular woman that took interest in him and wanted to write a story and she will print it in Detroit Free Press so I begin to let her come by her name was Mrs Dixion. I let her come by once or twice a week just to interview him and talk to him. Where he can communicate with them. And be comfortable but in the process of them coming these two big boxes also came inside these two boxes were medical papers College letters dating all the way back to 1989 I began to organize the letters by the dates and go look through the medical paperwork and I begin to look through his medical history and we found out things we hadn't even known me and my siblings as we read his medical history but one thing we found out we had three other siblings that we had no knowledge of, and they were much older than us. We never met them or we never knew them but his siblings did. so that was a blessing but at this time we were just concerned about our father so what I did I begin to send out for more medical records because some of the things that I read in the box I was looking at was major concern to me, some of the items I was looking at. I was concern because it said he was diagnosed with cancer in 2014 but we was not made aware of it until 2016 so that brought up a red flag then I looked in the other medical papers indicated to me that his hands have been broken and not repaired because he didn't give them permission. So then I begin to contact Richard handlon Correctional Facility and request for more medical paperwork because I felt as though I need to check deeper into this as my medical papers begin to come in I found out that our father was diagnosed with schizophrenia and paranoia I was aware that he dealt with depression but I didn't know it got to the point where it was that serious where he wasn't able to make his own decisions in the early stage. Of the diagnosis yes I found out in 2016 but from the papers I was reading his diagnosed started much earlier than 2016 the schizophrenia. so this became a little project for me because I did want to know as much information as I could and regards to his medical and what took place with him while being incarcerated in the meantime the Detroit Free Press will stop by once or twice a week take pictures talk to him to communicate with us and we consider it a blessing because he was gone for 33 years for $12 we had had individual from the Lansing parole board all the way to Ypsilanti did Tell us that he was not going to make it out of prison. But me and my husband made agreement the day before Christmas 2016,that we were going to trust God and stand on his word understand that some things only come by praying and fasting we all know that with man things are impossible but With God all things are possible so me and my husband begin to pray about the situation you pray according to

God's word we thanked him in advance, afterwards we thanked him as if it was already done. I have learned on this walk with God you have to believe it before you see it. the world tell you to see it then believe it .in God's kingdom is vice versa me and my husband made that agreement right around Christmas within 60 days he came home and we give all the glory to God, not man with all the medical papers that came after he came home dating from 1989 through 2016 we knew it can been nobody but God, these medical papers have doctors reports here are some of his medical conditions as a child was documented on them. so we begin to put them in order and we begin to let them take pictures of this information all of this became part of his interview we had made agreement to allow the Detroit Free Press to come by at least 4 times a month and watch us interact and communicate with our father. thank God my daughter Jessica had the experience of CNA and me myself I also was a caregiver in the past with my mother and my grandmother and now it's been going on two months now since our father's release between Outreach going to church working part time keeping up with our dad and I thank God for the nurses that was coming by. I began to notice my daughter she wasn't saying much she mostly was staying to herself but you know like I said earlier in the story multitasking miracles I called it an M&M I learn when serving God they'll be times that you're going to have to not only deal with your situation but you're going to have to deal with others too but that's what God strengthens us to do, and in helping others you helping yourself so I made up in my mind that on one of those weekends Saturdays Sundays and she's off work that I happen to have a talk with her but in the meantime I was just thanking God for the miracle that he had done I mostly was happy for my siblings because I had relationship with our dad in the past 8 years but neither one of them had seen him in over 20 years, I loved just watching him interact when they come by and watch movies sitting laughing talking it was really a blessing, but like I said we look straight ahead but God know what's around the corner.

A lot of times in life if you allow your mind to think on the problem more than the promise you will find yourself in a depressed state but the Bible says Philippians 4 verse 8 it tell us what to think on say it's finally my brother think on whatsoever things are true whatsoever things that are honest whatsoever things that are just whatsoever things that are pure whatsoever things that are lovely whatsoever things that are good report if there be any virtue and if there be any praise think on these things, when problems arise we have to elevate our mind right there get your mind off the problem and set it on the promise I find for me if you think on the problem more, some problems can get you in a depressed state but in the midst of the depression you have to find a praise there's something in your life you can praise God for and if you can't find nothing else just thank God for what he did sending you his dear son Jesus .making a way out of no way and as you begin to lift him up and give God the praise and as you begin to magnify his name he will turn your midnight to Daylight. as I sit here and I think about prayer it takes my mind to my Bishop Bishop Eddie Watson he is a praying man and he wrote a book called prayer it's bigger than you are and his wife First Lady Barbara Watson play a key role in me and my husband's life. But for me its personal because my mother and father are decease. They are my spiritual mother and father and in his book he wrote about prevailing and persistent prayer and it's located on page 21 in his book, this is what really stuck out to me he said successful prayer requires a persistent spirit there will be problems obstacles and conditions that seem as if they will never be corrected but out love for God and our confidence in his word causes us to hang on when it appears that there is nothing to hang onto. Then you say we must be encouraged through the word and know that God will deliver and help us and right there was the key for me. when problems arise in situations occur we run away from God but we need to run to him why because it's his word that encourages us. and that will deliver us to help us get through every situation Psalms 121 says it best I will lift up my eyes to the Hills from whence cometh my help .and that's why I say in the midst of bipolar disorder in the midst of whatever your situation is in the midst of you hurt in the midst of your pain and the health condition in the midst of your relationship good or bad you submit your situation in that spot but whatever the condition find a praise. For me it was bipolar disorder I had to find a praise and in me praising him in the situation I was in. I praise my way out. and God snatch me out and look how many miracles he performed after I came out of Darkness into His Marvelous Light. the same God that did it for me will do it for anybody but you got to want him more than anything. you got to know your way out is going in you stay in the word in him (God) Acts chapter 17 verse 28 says its in him we live and move and have our being, whatever you do you got to be true to yourself, there's nothing wrong with telling on yourself. God already Knows and that makes it better because he's the one got to help you fix it and he already knows what it's going to take while we thinking about it he already. Has took care of it just waiting on you to be truthful. John chapter 8 verse 32 say ye shall no the truth and the truth will set you free. Well I said earlier I was going to have a talk with my daughter and I did I thank god she works she take care of herself she has her own transportation come to find out she was staying to herself cause after I talked to her she confirmed to me and told me that she was pregnant and I couldn't get upset because she did the unexpected she graduated she walked across the stage she had her own job and transportation and finances and she was over 21 but then I looked at it as another miracle because I told you early in the story when she was 4 years old she had a bone development issue and one of her legs and she had over 10 surgical. Procedures so from developing as a child we was not sure if she could have children. From the bone discrepancy so they didn't know whether she was going to be able to have children because of the condition so we had a moment and we talked she cried we cried I encouraged her because. That's what we here to do for our kids I learned with my children they got to make their own mistakes and the enemy will use them to slow down your process if u let him, he will use individuals that are close to you and the ones that you love, justs to slow down progress, but you got to have a made up mind that whatever the situation is there's nothing too hard for God. I just begin to pray for her and tell her to be encouraged we had our weekly. Talks and we became. Closer also. But as I said earlier we still work and do god will when it comes to the ministry you can't let situation and circumstances get you in a place where you can not service God. I told her I love her and she knows who I am, also know what I do and what I stand for, so I still have to go to church I still have to do Outreach Bible study and I still have to do the work in the ministry. That's one thing about me and my husband. We try Not to stop. Things that start in the ministry we didn't want to be the type of individuals that start something and stop so I continue to let the Detroit Free Press come by the house. Now we were just coming up on two months and they were still making their regular visits taking pictures. Our dad even had a parole officer that would stop by.

CHAPTER 9
Say It to See It

I don't know what they expected him to do but I guess that's just how the state Authority operate. Anyway I begin to notice a few changes when it came to our father he wasn't talking as much and this is around the first week in April he wasn't saying much I found that when I did come in the room with him he would want to know about his mother he'll be asking me about her and that was a area he stayed in denial with even though his mama had passed in 2011 and he was informed he didn't want to accept it. dealing with that situation I was caught like between a rock and a hard place, because when he asked me about his mother and I began to tell him she's no longer with us he would get upset and he would get frustrated and get angry so I plan on avoiding the subject but one night I went to his room to check on him and he was talking to himself and I asked him who was he talking to and he said his mother, so I didn't have much to say about that I just pray for him when I did not go to sleep sometimes at night I began to talk to my siblings about it to let them know what was going on the nurses that were coming by. The nurses indicated to me that this is a stage people go through when they are declining in health but anyway I just continue to stay in Christ pray read, make his breakfast his lunch and dinner whenever me and my husband went out to do work in the community we had to let the kids. Know. We also informed. Them of the nurse. Schedule. Because. She continue to come by twice a week the Detroit Free Press still stop by and took pictures sat with us we kept them informed then one early morning I got up had to be like 5 a.m. and I went in to change a DVD player because he like to watch The Five Heartbeats he wasn't saying much he always wanted water or juice to drink through the night so I got him some juice I look at our daddy I cut the light on I cut the DVD player back on because whenever I go to the bathroom I can always hear him because the bathroom was right next to his room, so I went back to my room and I just laid there it seem like the longest. Hour I could not sleep for about an hour and a half I got up at 7:30 to get his breakfast ready went to the bathroom brush my teeth wash my face here it is around April 17 and the week before he passed I had contacted my siblings and told them stop by and see how he was doing and they did, because I did take in consideration what the direct care worker was saying, about the different stages individuals go thru, and the nurses were more experienced in this area then i was, I also had contact his siblings that week even his brother had came up to visit our dad, his younger brother named Gregory and his wife came, from out of town around the end of March, And I thank God for that, because 3 weeks later I get up to go to the bathroom early morning April 24th 7:30 a.m. I brush my teeth wash my face because I got up to get breakfast ready and as I cut the water on in the bathroom and I cut it off I didn't hear no breathing no shallow breathing no movement anything so, I went in the bedroom and I said Dad dad I call his name like three times cut the light on he looked like he was sleep. I put my hand on his chest where his heart is I didn't feel anything his body was kind of warm, picked up his wrist for a pulse I didn't get none then I begin to call the nurse she indicated to me that they were going to call doctor then I called my siblings to come over they were about 15 minutes away they were right around the corner, his body was still a little warm by the time my siblings arrive within 7 minutes 5 minutes later the nurse came in the house and walked in the room., and she came out and she pronounced him deceased then the nurse got on the phone and begin to make calls at that moment my sister and brother it was like me holding babies all over again I had one on the right and on the left I think my husband must have felt bad for me because he help me with my sister this was a trying time this is one of those situations that you can't look at the problem you got to stand on the promise and then believe whatever the situation is God going to fix it, My heart went out for my siblings little more then myself because it was like they had lost him twice. I think for me I was mostly numb it was like I didn't really have no emotion it happen so quick but this is the way it was with my mom and after everything was over everybody was gone and when it get quiet and you all alone that's when everything set in. I knew that this is going to be one of those trying times but I still had to keep my focus after the coroner came in the nurse left, my siblings they were really sad and down I begin to tell them that we could just thank God, and be grateful for the time and the memories that God gave us with our father especially my siblings since they hadn't seen him in close to 20 years. I think we sat at home for the rest of the day thinking and talking about him eating Kentucky Fried Chicken looking at The Five Heartbeats and watching Andy Griffith these were the memories that we were left to share and I thank God for that yes we were hurting but as my husband always say things can be worse, now I knew we had things set up that we had to face funeral expenses and different things like that I thank God for my oldest children especially Jimmy and Jamaal and James helping with the obituary. A lot of arrangements had to be made but I just knew that God will get us through it one thing I did thank God for, I can say God

- Did It Again because even though our father passed away we did have a say so in this part of his life and we did get to spend it with him. God did what I asked him to. I asked him to bring him home with us so if he did pass he would pass with loving family members around him now as I said before the Detroit Free Press continue to still come by. I made the call to them. The following day and explain what took place in his passing Detroit. Free press writer begin to ask me if they could come by and record the funeral services I gave them permission to take a few pictures they had been with us all this time. So the funeral service was a process I said they can take part in, also as we begin to plan the funeral service. Much work had to be done. Obituaries. Order of service. Where the family. Going to eat I thank god I was affiliated with a church, my pastor. Did the eulogy. I thank god for these three women of god one was a Mrs Carissa Watson. she is married. Earl Watson. Carissa and her siblings the Collins family is a well known family in the community that was well respected, and our dad childhood friends she also has a sister name Delphine and she married a Mr Holman they were a blessing to me also. They new our father before I existed. And these were the two women. He always talked about when ever I went to visit him while incarcerated. I didn't no at that time that 20 years later When I turn my life over to god. later I ended up in there church. Home god knows what to do and when to do it and one day I was telling someone. Who our dad was at church and my god she new so much about our father sis Carissa and her sister Delphine they even new the dog he had and the name of the dog was rex. As a teenager it was truly a blessing. To here things about our father we never knew. So I thank god for being a all knowing god. he always. Mentioned. His childhood friends and another young lady. well known in the community. Known for helping others before. Helping herself this women told me about. A man that will save me and set me free and deliver me she led me to Christ evangelist

- boone. These women. Were a blessing. To me at a time when it seem. Like the world was on my. Shoulders and also sis Cheryl and her husband bro Larry. Cheryl has a beautiful spirit. And she always had a encouraging word to say. and a evangelist byrd. A awesome women of god. All of these women participated in our dad funeral. They were really a blessing. To me At our dad funeral. So after everything. Was over it all went well. We all had to pull together. With information. That was need for services such as his mom and dad school attendance. Ect. Thats where his siblings. Came in, like I say god no what to do and when to do it while you trying to figure it out God has already worked it out. so After.

The funeral. I continue to need more answers in regards to his health so not only did I have the medical records that he brought home I begin to order a number a medical release information and I thank God for my son James because he was such a blessing ordering medical records getting information that was needed so we can begin to speak to someone to find out why was our father diagnosed with this condition and sat in prison for over 2 years without getting treatment. I understand that it was going to be a process but I just sat back and thank God. For Matthew 19 and 26 with man it is impossible but with God all things are possible. even though our father passed it was sad. but I was glad he made it home I told my siblings, I give God all the glory for that truly I understand the saying if it had not been for the Lord that was on my side I don't know what I would have done. I thank God for the Memories he gave me and my siblings because up until that point we had none. That's one thing about our grandma she always used to tell us when one life goes out another one comes in. my Grandma had a saying for everything I guess you can call them sticky quotes she would tell us the grass is greener on the other side, why buy the cow when you can get the milk for free, and don't cry over spilled milk. Don't go through life too fast you'll forget to smell the flowers don't lay down with dogs you get up with fleas. Everything That Glitters Is Not Gold. me I will add my own it was the enemy can paint ugly picture but when you know the artist you can always change of scenery I called them sticky quotes I find that things in life can cause you to feel depressed feel down you can be diagnosed with a depression condition but in the midst of it all and the mist of bipolar disorder or whatever your condition is. Meaning you fill in the blank because we all know what we struggle with it's no secret from God he knows all too. but you have to find a praise there's always a reason to praise God there is always a reason to lift him up. the word of God tells us in the presence of the Lord is fullness of joy. and what praise will do it will set the platform to usher in God's presence, and I made up in my mind that I need God I can't make it without him I've learned to tell my problems about my God and not my God about my problems because he already knows. when I think about praise it reminds me of the donkey the story where the donkey fell in the hole and the master decided the donkey was old so he was going to cover the donkey up with dirt so as he kept on piling the dirt on the Donkey. The dirt would land on the donkey's back and he would shake the dirt off his back, and pack it under his feet .and take a step up and the more he continued To shake the dirt off and step up he ended up stepping right out the hole so whenever you praise and lift up your holy hands you shaking the dirt off and as you lift up your hands and praise God the dirt fall under your feet and when you continue to do it whatever the problem whatever holding you back your praise will shake the dirt off your back. So we can pack it under your feet, and cause you to rise above your situation and bring you out. just like the Donkey that donkey had to keep packing that dirt until it lifted him up out of that hole just as the

CHAPTER 10
God Did It

onkey had to keep packing the dirt underneath him to be lifted up out of the hole, we have to give God a praise so praise will escort us into his presence So we can be. lifted up and out of what ever situation trying to keep us bound. I thank God for the many blessings that he has bestowed on me and my family and I thank God for all the memories especially when it comes to our father but as my grandmother always told us when one life goes out another one comes in. I hadn't talked to my daughter in a while because she was working and her job required her to work 12 hours a day but I knew of her situation and I would just take out time every Saturday to have a mom and daughter day so we can talk, and as time went on the months went pass and when I looked around I started going to the doctor with her after we got past the hurt pain and crying, I just continue to encourage her .now it is coming up on our pastors appreciation time and everybody always makes plans around this time of the year to do something special for our pastors so that was first priority this is where everybody do their fundraising and getting money together and finances together to show their appreciation for their pastors so much work needed to be done. So after September pass me and Jessica's father decided that we were going to sit down and have a family discussion how she was going to deal with the pregnancy of the child we were very happy for her because I said earlier we were not even sure she could conceive, she had decided that she was going to work till The Bitter End but we all know we can all decide one way but our way may not be God's so as she begin to come up close on her due date she started dealing with health problems with her back her legs and the doctors started getting concerned about her health so what we begin to do, me and my husband as I said before we don't like to start and stop anything, we decided that we would have to take turns sometime he may go out and pass out flyers I may go to the doctor with her or we will schedule the doctor's appointments around Outreach times but God worked it all out I believe she got down to the last month December

2017 and she had to stop work because it got too difficult for her, and that's where we had to step in and start assist her but even in the midst of it all you have to refuse to let anything separate you from God Romans 8 verse 35 because through it all God was going to have to be the one to help us get through it, at this time it got kind of difficult being that the majority of the family members was deceased and her father and I had to do a lot of running a lot of errands. Strategizing. So we can stay on track and thanking god for his strength, the young man her fiance came up here he was from New Jersey he would start coming twice a month to sit with her but after she delivered the baby he begin to come more frequently but until then me and her dad had to step up to the plate, and her younger brother James he was always there for. His sister regardless of what they went through, and this was the month of December this is the Christmas month, this is the time when everybody is running around getting gifts getting set up for the holiday we didn't know whether she was going to have a Christmas baby or New Year's baby we was just praying for just a healthy child we did find out early what she was going to have which was a boy. so me and my husband decided to name him Messiah with her permission and it was such a coincidence because the young man which was my grandchild father he was all the way in New Jersey and came up with the same name so that was confirmation for us and with everything going on around the holidays this is the time when you do a lot of thinking about your loved ones especially the ones that is no longer here, but I still give glory to God just for the opportunity and the time that we had. With our dear father, now New Year's is right around the corner and you know how everyone every beginning of the new year they make New Year's resolutions decide New Beginnings things are going to change but as I said earlier the only thing I try to keep in my life is Jesus because when you make New Year's resolutions they always get broken and the majority of the time they're never fulfilled so it's best to just make life-changing decisions and stick with them and stay in

Christ with everything that was going on me and my husband still had to attend Outreach programs and this is the time of year there's a lot of Christmas programs also so what we did was something special we decided when we went to the convalescent home this year we would take a lot of blankets and socks and packages to the elderly people. this is something that we tried to do each year with the help of the Outreach team at our church now that Christmas is over and we coming into the new year you know as they always say fresh start new beginning Jessica was set up to go to the doctor after January 5th her feet begin to swell with fluid so they took her off of work early how many of you know that when a situation arise we all know the battle is in your mind, because what he will do he will start trying to plant seeds telling you negative thoughts and this is where you can't come half-cocked you got to come fully loaded with the word of God. you have to do just what Jesus did in Matthew 4 and verse 4 he told him what was written. Now you operating in Warfare your weapons for warfare is the word, and 2nd Corinthians chapter 10 and verse 4 and 5. also. Joshua chapter 1 verse 8. this is how I try to combat problems the majority of the time, because regardless of what you go through the enemy can paint an ugly picture but like I say when you know the artist you can always change the scenery. as time progress the doctors had considered inducing her labor but me and my husband we just stayed in prayer they had her coming in monitoring the baby at least once a week but we just choose to believe God. And we demonstrated that belief by what we did. Prayed about it then we thank god for the results. And took care of gods business and we begin to see the manifestation of what we were praying for. as I said before yes problems are going to rise but they don't have to get inside of you if you stay in Jesus the problems will stay on the outside meaning that we need to keep our focus on Jesus reminds me of the story of Peter in the Book of Matthew as he walked on the water and he called out to Jesus Master if it is you to tell me to come but one thing about Peter he was boldest out of all disciples he stepped out there on the water, and as he begin to walk he was fine as long as he kept his focus and his eyesight on Jesus but he got distracted and he begin to sink and that lets me know that in life we going to have distractions and we have to keep our eyes on Jesus because if we don't those distractions will cause us to sink stumble and fall and even if you do fall or stumble get yourself up dust yourself off and have your conversation with Jesus and get right back into the race, so as we made our trip to U of M Hospital and they begin to monitor Jessica on January 12th 2018 after 20 hours of labor they gave her a C-section and she delivered her baby boy name Messiah I give all the glory to God. and I learn this here that whatever you go through in life you always going to have ups and downs you always going to have situations and circumstances you have to face your going to have to choose to believe God. you going to have to stay in faith stay in the word stay in prayer because one thing I found out that faith that's contaminated. Meaning. Allowing doubt to come in this will open the door to fear so whatever you go through keep your eyes on Jesus and always know in the midst of. Any negative situation weather its depression hurt anger. Jealousy frustrations what ever is hindering you slowing down progress there's always a praise that whatever we go through in life we still owe him a praise and the word of God tells us in psalm 68 let God arise and his enemies be scattered Thank you Jesus. this book is dedicated to anyone that have ever felt lost to anyone that's ever felt alone to anyone that felt as if no one is there or no one cares. I come to tell you that one out of every five adults and one out of every four young adults will experience mental illness disorder 90% of suicide occurs, through mental illness, mental illness is not prejudiced it doesn't care who it hits depression does not care about race or color, they'll be times you feel hopeless there will be times you feel alone they'll be times you feel as if no one is there and no one cares but this is why Jesus died to set us free .yes there are doctors available and they're also counselors available to and no this we all have problems but it's how we deal with the problems that makes the difference .this condition includes our emotional and psychological and social well-being depression can affects how we think feel and act as we cope with life it interferes with how we handle stress and relate to others and also the choices that we make. Mental illness is a serious disorder that can affect your thinking and your mood and your life but I come to tell you yes they have Prozac yes they have lithium celexa Thorazine yes they have Zoloft yes they have a Risperdal for racing thoughts and I can keep going on and on the list is never-ending. And I have tried them all from. Electric shock treatment to the medication but I come to tell you the best medication that you can take is three doses of the word of God daily and don't just take it part of the time take it all the time Joshua 1:8 says to meditate in my word day and night it does not just say in the day only, and it does not just say the night it says day and night to make your way prosperous and have good success the same god that delivered me can deliver anybody all you got to do is want it and believe. One thing I found out when it comes to God's word that the word of God will keep you but you have to meditate in that word even when you doing good stay in God's word because it's his word that is going to strengthen you. Separate yourself from negative situation negative people work on you getting delivered then when you are strong enough, Come be a blessing to others because you can't help others when you a mess amen. No it's his word that's going to keep you, John 15 verse 3 tells us we are clean by his word one of my favorite scriptures is Psalms 115 verse 14. And also job 22 verse 28, I meditated on those, scripture for the past 7 years and believe me just about everything I've asked God to do it is now come to pass and I was in position. Doing God's will and keeping myself in position to be used by god. I thank God for our son James for being the writer of this book, my daughter Jessica, my sons Jimmy and Jamaal and step-children Nikyta and Paul and also my two siblings Montez and Niecy and also all our grandchildren. I thank God for my husband Paul Wilson he always use encouraging words

To Say when you think it's bad always remember it could be worse I found out in life we all going to have storms we have to encounter but the storm can be on the outside it don't have to be in you .and some people. Experience. Storms in different. Levels such as light rain thunderstorms. Some seem like. Hurricane. And tsunami but if you can just keep your focus on Jesus in spite of your situation not on what you going through. You say how? For me it goes back to Colossians chapter 3 verse 2 set your mind on what's above and not on what's on this earth, and key is to keep it set, for me to keep it set is understanding that whatever the situation I am in God is the one got to bring me out I can't do it whether it's good or bad yes God has to fix it. he has given us everything. We need to rise above any situation that keeping us from getting where we need to be in God .and stay connected by any means necessary this is the conclusion I had to come to., problems are going to come and there will be times these problems will get you in a place where you feel like you depressed but in the midst of your depression there's always a praise in the midst of your hurt there's always a praise in the midst of your confusion there's always a praise in the midst of your loneliness there's always a praise when you can't see your way there is always a praise whatever your situation is you fill in the blank but there is always a praise, because the word of God lets us know that the Praises belong to God. Psalms 34 says I will bless the Lord at all times and his Praises shall continually be in my mouth in the midst of depression give God the praise. and the praise will rise you above your situation or your circumstances and my God inhabits the Praises of his people according to Psalms 22 verse 3 what I found out is praise will confuse the enemy praise is defined as an expression of or approval commodation elaboration praise is the invitation of God's arrival praise is the connection of communication between your prayer life and your standard with God every time you lift your hands and surrender to God. Satan is saying dang I thought I had you. but you still have your hands raised giving God glory and thanking him praise honors God according to Luke 11 Jesus taught us to begin prayers with praise in order to honor and glorify God. Psalms 29 tells us to give glory to God praise helps us focus on God. Psalms 22 verse 3 say God inhabits the Praises of his people praise helps us to know God. it helps us to focus on his character and his attributes praise breaks the enemy's oppression in Acts 16 Paul and Silas praise God and the prison doors where open their chains fell off, the Jailer and there families were saved and most important praise confuses the forces of evil the power of praise in the battle is shown and 2nd Chronicles 20 story of jehoshaphat Psalms 8 verse 2. Psalms 149 verse 5 through 9 praise helps us to focus on God and realize our need for God. And this turns the battle over to God when we do this God brings victory this makes praise and prayer dependency on God great weapons in the spiritual battle. Before I even go into prayer these are steps to remember step one pray with a clean heart and pure hands, Psalms 24 verse 4 we must be able to approach God but to do that we need to operate in Psalms 24 verse 4 Step 2 Proverbs 28 verse 13 whoever conceals their sins does not prosper but the one who confesses and renounces them finds Mercy. step 3 proverbs 3 verse 5 through 6 trust in the Lord with all thy heart and lean not to your own understanding in all thy ways acknowledge Him and He will direct your path. And step four Hebrews 11 verse 6 without faith it's impossible to please God. And step 5 1st Thessalonians 5 Verse 18 in everything give thanks for this is God's will for you in Christ Jesu.s this book is dedicated to anyone that understand there is power in Praise and understand Psalms 34 and verse 1, I thank God for my husband paul Wilson my brother Montez and sister Niecy my children Jimmy Jamaal James Jessica my step children Paul and Nikyta grandchildren godchildren and stepchildren I pray that someone would be encouraged delivered and set free and a special thanks to the writer of the book my son James Brooks Brown and I give all the glory to God. I don't say god is the head of my life, he is all of my life and I thank god for letting me be a vessel for his use I love you Lord you truly are friend that sticks closer than a brother.

* Dear reader I want you to understand how powerful praise is when you can learn to praise God in the midst of the situation in spite of whatever is going on in spite of whatever is trying to destroy you or annoy you then you are ready to see the hand of God move in your life you'll be able to say Psalms 34 I will bless the Lord at all times and his Praises that shall continually be in my mouth not only should you say it you are to live it and be it Psalms 150 verse 6 says let everything that has breath praise the Lord the. table of contents

I would also like to thank every mother I have encountered in my life that spoke a word in my life that saw the best in me & prayed that it would manifest it in my life. From my grandma Juanita Warren, mother Patricia Brooks, mother in law Flora O'day, grandmother Delilah Brooks my spiritual mother 1st lady Barbara Watson and anyone I may missed thank you & God Bless I love you and appreciate you And thank u lord for blessing me to be a blessing to others. And I thank God for my God nephew Orlando he had a beautiful spirit but passed away june 27th 2021 he also suffered from depression in early 2000 along with Rochelle P she passed away also as so many others are suffering today. Special thanks to Elder Spratt and Prophetess Spratt a blessed man and woman of God that always gave me and my husband a encouraging word. I Also thank God for my jobs Rpc Rehab kohls and Arro maintenance my jobs they worked with me and was so understanding thru the trials I endured and God delivered me, and especially thanks to my supervisor Mr bank and the employees at Rpc

A special thanks to Manny at Pac n Parcel in Ypsilanti Michigan, a very supportive young man who always gave me an encouraging word. You are truly a blessing and definitely an asset in the community

PRAYER THOUGHTS

PRAYER THOUGHTS

PRAYER THOUGHTS

PRAYER THOUGHTS

Printed in the United States
by Baker & Taylor Publisher Services